ELDERCARE

ISBN 1552123502

FORTHCOMING FROM GEORGE H. WEBER

Novels

Box Car
Abide With Me

Short Stories

In Pursuit of Altruism

ELDERCARE

A CLINICAL PRIMER

FOR VOLUNTEERS

George H. Weber

Copyright © 2000 by George H. Weber.

Printed in Canada

Canadian Cataloguing in Publication Data

Weber, George H.
   Eldercare

   Includes bibliographical references and index.
   ISBN 1-55212-350-2

   1. Aged--Care.   2. Caregivers.   3. Aging--Psychological aspects.   I. Title.
HV1451.W42 2000   362.6   C00-910218-3

TRAFFORD

This book was published on-demand in cooperation with Trafford Publishing.
On-demand publishing is a unique process and service of making a book available for retail
sale to the public taking advantage of on-demand manufacturing and Internet marketing.
On-demand publishing includes promotions, retail sales, manufacturing, order fulfilment,
accounting and collecting royalties on behalf of the author.

Suite 6E, 2333 Government St., Victoria, B.C. V8T 4P4, CANADA
Phone   250-383-6864   Toll-free   1-888-232-4444 (Canada & US)
Fax   250-383-6804   E-mail   sales@trafford.com
Web site   www.trafford.com   trafford publishing is a division of trafford holdings ltd.
Trafford Catalogue #00-0014   www.trafford.com/robots/00-0014.html

10   9   8   7   6   5   4   3   2

Permission to Quote

Permission granted by:

NATIONAL MENTAL HEALTH ASSOCIATION

> To reprint its public statement on "Medication for Mental Health." The section primarily concerned with children was deleted

RUSSELL SAGE FOUNDATION

> To quote from Mary Richmond, *Friendly Visiting Among the Poor.*

Table of Contents

Foreword

With the aging of the population, the demographic composition of the country is simultaneously changing. Along with the growth of the older population have been shifts in the social structure. Families are smaller and more mobile than in previous decades and the majority of women are employed outside of the home. Consequently, the ability of the informal network to provide support and help to frail relatives is often restricted Yet, frailty connotes dependency and often a pressing need for assistance. Such assistance should not be limited to professionals. Volunteers can play major roles in meeting the needs of many of these older persons both in the community and in institutions.

Although good intentions and goodwill provide a framework for this support, in themselves they are not sufficient to adequately address the many issues involved in care. Through its focus on educating and training persons so that their efforts and involvement have a maximum impact on the older people they seek to help, this book fills a noticeable gap in the literature related to volunteering.

The book addresses both the general problems affecting elderly persons in long term care, as well as specific strategies that volunteers can use to help them deal with these problems. These are clearly illustrated through case examples of situations commonly encountered in long term care settings, along with specific suggestions of how to work with them.

Volunteering can be extremely rewarding, but it can also be frustrating. Such frustration may cause many to cease their volunteer involvement. Hopefully, the material in this unique book will help to ensure that the volunteer experience remains a positive one in which persons continue to grow and develop as they simultaneously enhance the lives of the older persons with whom they work.

– Carole Cox, Ph.D.
Associate Professor
Graduate School of Social Service
Fordham, University

Acknowledgments

I am very appreciative of Jay Kenny, DSW and Suzanne Lord, MSW for giving me an opportunity to work as a volunteer in the Public Guardianship Program, Aging and Disability Services of the Department of Health and Human Services, Montgomery County, Maryland, and for their insightful instruction and sound counsel in that effort. Also, I appreciate critical reading of an earlier version of this manuscript and positive suggestions by Mary Scantlebury, M.A. and Mary Ann Llewellyn. Also acknowledged is Ms. O, a colleague who has chosen to remain anonymous. She generously shared a number of case histories with me (although, to maintain consistency in the book, the volunteer is referred to as masculine). Susan P. Fossett, word processor of the highest order and thoughtful advisor, is greatly appreciated for her contribution, and thanks to Cynthia MacGregor for thoughtful and exacting editorial advice and copy editing. Last, and most important, I am indebted to the clients whom I got to know in the course of volunteering.

Introduction

This book was stimulated by Mary Richmond's classic, *Friendly Visiting Among the Poor* (1918). Richmond organized most of that work in terms of the poor persons' roles: head of family, employee, husband and father, wife as homemaker, and children as students and dependents. Some of her presentation was more general; for example, she included topics on the family's health and recreation and its spending and saving, the principles of effective poor relief, and the relation of the church to the poor.

In this framework, Richmond recommended a number of counseling techniques: using tact and good will, a kindly spirit, sympathy, earnestness and dignity; generating new interests; and cheering in the joys and opinions of clients and sympathizing with their sorrows. Indeed, she urged the visitor to share the poor person's entire outlook on life. She reasoned that the friendly visitor's best work preparation stemmed from her own life experience and was rooted in her empathy and commitment.

This book attempts to emulate Richmond's work, particularly her: (1) addressing, "What do you say when facing a client?" "How do you say it?" "For what purpose?"; (2) incisive case histories to exemplify the text; and (3) careful observation to distinguish surface behavior from underlying dynamics.

However, the work is considerably different from Richmond's classic. First, it concerns the elderly, not the poor. Moreover, it focuses on the psychosocial problems of the elderly, not on their income maintenance problems, though many elderly are poor. Second, it is psychologically more subtle than Richmond's direct, persuasive approach to influence her clients. Also the current work is not concerned with the client's social class strivings, whereas Richmond pressed middle class values onto her clients, which she thought were in their best interest.

The current book presents the major skills required in monitoring as well as psychologically engaging elderly persons, especially those in long-term care. Elementary skills for the beginner as well as some advanced ones for the more seasoned practitioner are covered. Skills that address the elderly person's current concerns in the context of her earlier experiences—especially unresolved problematic experiences—are given particular emphasis. The elderly persons of concern include the frail and debilitated because of strokes and early dementias, the mentally disturbed, including those who are paranoid, and the elderly who are fully intact yet suffer from the effects of loss, isolation, and despair.

What can be achieved is limited by what the elderly person brings, her psychological and genetic strengths and her social supports. Also, a variety of goals may be sought, ranging from limited ones (such as reducing the client's psychological strain and anxiety through short-term intervention) to more substantial goals (including the ventilation and resolution of current and associated earlier life problems, especially as the earlier problems causally relate to the immediate ones). The book:

- Describes the qualities necessary to pursue volunteer work;
- Considers the population of concern and its needs;
- Gives you helpful information on how to initiate an interview, and how to continue working with a client. That is, specific techniques are described and examples are given;
- Tells how and when to make referrals;
- Suggests how to work with families and other personnel involved in a client's case;
- Helps you understand the scope of your task through many examples of interviews with clients;
- Indicates how to use supervision;
- Provides effective tips for coping with the stress that is a natural part of volunteering;
- Considers standards of ethical behavior for you.

The lack of family involvement in most of the cases cited in the book is because there either wasn't one, or they were unable or unwilling to contribute. Most of the elderly considered are residents in a nursing home. A notation is made when such is not the case.

This book will be of greatest interest to volunteers working with the elderly, especially those volunteers with clinical concerns; that is, concerns for the elderly's feelings—good and bad—their worries, fears, hopes, aspirations, daily activities, struggles and relationships. Supervisors of volunteers may find the book helpful in guiding volunteers in their development. Finally, professionals may find the material stimulating in program planning.

I
Being a Volunteer

Being a volunteer working with the elderly should stem from your humanistic commitment, including passion and will, to preserve the dignity of older people, to maximize their quality of life and to help them resolve their problems, to the extent that such is possible.

Irrespective of your educational preparation, you must have a genuine concern about the physical, psychological, social and spiritual welfare of aged persons, including those who are infirm and lacking in physical mobility and mental sharpness. Furthermore, you must be able to identify the elderly person's interests, concerns and preoccupations, draw these out with patience and compassion, work out personal problems and continue through resistances, deficits in functioning and discouraging events. That it is hard, demanding work is clear, particularly the emotional aspects of the work, which may become burdensome. The elderly person may become progressively more incapacitated, begin to—and actually—die, leaving you struggling with your own emotions: anxiety, sadness, anger and frustration. Yet, hopefully the satisfaction of having done a good humanitarian deed will usually override negative feelings.

Your role also involves monitoring and acting on behalf of the elderly and advocating their interests to those who officially make decisions about their situation—spouses, family members, guardians and officials of care-providing agencies. You must be in contact with these persons to give them information and to get help from them.

Orienting Point of View

You should have information, at least at an elementary level, about aging, including factors that play into personal stress and feelings of despair and frustration. Further, information about support centers, group homes, nursing homes and assisted living will add to your background. Motivation to advance your knowledge as well as your skill will help in all areas of your performance. You must listen and think about the meaning of what the elderly person says and does. Through time these expressions will show the pattern of the elderly person's life—challenges, problems and successes—and how she has dealt with them, and how you might help her. The client's physical status, especially her medical condition, should be known to you. Might she have cancer? If so, what kind, and in what phase is it, and what is the prognosis? Similar considerations apply in regard to a heart condition, Alzheimer's disease, mental illness and all other mental or physical conditions.

If the client requires incidental services, you must decide whether you will provide them; for example, transportation, clothing purchases and so on. If you decide to provide such services, you must decide how much you can reasonably do. Given the humanitarian tendency to overly commit oneself at the beginning of a relationship, you must think through what you can realistically do—what you can live with—and make that known to the person in charge of the case and to the client.

Psychological Work

The immediate and continuing circumstance of facing the elderly person requires you to assess how she feels, that is, her attitude and outlook—whether she is amiable and good natured, matter-of-fact and even tempered, or hostile and testy.

In a casual, informal way, you must encourage the elderly person to talk and express herself. Further, you must listen and grapple with what she says and does not say to understand her thoughts, memories and feelings. That is, you stimulate the elderly person to talk about herself, her current circumstances, including that which preoccupies and troubles her. You also encourage her to bring her earlier life experience to the fore, as such is appropriate. Through careful sifting and sorting, you may begin to see connections between earlier and current events, and you must try ever so skillfully to help the elderly person see and appreciate them as well, perhaps not immediately but as time progresses. The immediate objective is to initiate a relationship and develop a pattern of working together.

The longer-term objective, especially if the elderly person brings distressing problems into the conversation, is to consider the immediate problem for its connection to possible earlier ones. Further, the mulling over of the earlier experiences seeks to ease the current distress.

Since the elderly person tends to reminisce, you will find ample opportunity to help her explore the pattern of her early and more recent experiences and gain an integrated view of her life. If, however, the plan is to concentrate on daily matters and any immediate reality problem the client has, you must stay with that. Such a limited strategy may be in order if the client's problem is not "deep-seated," or, on the other hand, is too shaky to undertake anything emotionally upsetting. Even if you plan a longer-term relationship, you should limit the initial scope of your inquiry until you get a full view of the client's problems and her strengths.

In the course of the client's talking, she is likely to avoid, deny and otherwise hamper the process of discovery and perhaps hamper the resolution of the very problems she complains about. She does not do this to hinder progress or be obstinate, but to maintain her interpretation of events and her sense of balance, and to avoid painful emotions. However, if you are able to help her through her resistance with reassurance and support, she may be able to consider the problems fully.

However, you will face different types of clients. For example, the person may have speech and mental problems and therefore cannot verbalize, at least not very understandably; or the client may be antagonistic, uncooperative, perhaps paranoid and won't talk. In the former instance—the person with speech and conceptual difficulties—you may communicate with the client by attentively "reading" her concerns, empathizing with them and perhaps animating her expressions. This all means you must sustain exacting contact with the client, and study her animation, body language, and any verbalizations she may offer. Further, you must repeat back to her what you understand of what she has said. This is all done in the context of what she previously expressed, either in the current interview or in earlier ones. The idea is to build meaning into what she tries to communicate and to sustain the relationship.

If the client is antagonistic, the safest procedure is one of care and reassurance while calmly probing for the seat of the antagonism. Your calmness aims to ease the anger yet keep the point of "what's the matter" in focus. It is difficult to predict what might follow. The person may remain silent or deny any antagonism, in which instance you may wait a few moments, then ask further about her feeling, perhaps in a word or two. Or the person may respond very quickly to your first inquiry, even explode. If that response follows, be sure to handle it with ease and be sure she has her full say. If the client is at all amenable, including after an emotional outburst, you may empathize with her discontent, explore it, and work with her on it—being careful not to get entangled in a no-win argument. Not all engagements with the elderly are maneuvers—moves by you to help the client express herself and to put her more closely in touch with herself. Even watching TV together is appropriate, especially if the client is watching TV at the time you enter the situation and she is "glued" to the screen, or if she has limited ability to think reflectively because of a dementia, is exceptionally frail or has some other serious impairment. Such activity may seem non-clinical, yet it may be especially meaningful and supportive to the client. Minimally, in such circumstances, the client has your presence, interest and companionship, which are substantial in themselves. At other times of little activity by the client, you might ask her questions about her activities, engage in easy conversation and indulge in peaceful silence.

Monitoring Work

While you are positively disposed toward the elderly person, you also must maintain an objective, "diagnostic" eye on her condition. Clients are often frail and fragile, and thereby easily subject to deterioration. Hence, they must be monitored carefully. It is a special task. You, obviously, do not stand in the place of a physician, nurse, public health official or social worker unless you are one. However, you stand as an astute and sensitive observer with normal expectations, judgments and the common sense of a mature person in daily life. Any special training will serve you well. At any rate, you can be expected to note whether the physical capacities of the elderly person have dropped noticeably since your last call; whether the elderly person has any unexplained or implausibly explained injuries; whether the elderly person appears dehydrated, malnourished, unkempt or dirty; whether the elderly person is withdrawn, confused, depressed, agitated, irrational or regressed. Moreover, you should note the quality of the care setting, and the attitude and diligence of its staff.

The possibility of a frail client's condition worsening must be foremost in your consideration. On the other hand, her prospects for improving must also be kept in mind; for example, after having been moved from a chaotic living situation to a nurturing one.

Receptivity May Vary

The receptivity of elderly persons to you varies, depending on their psychological state, the briefing they get about your visiting and your skill. Usually you and the client will receive information about each other from the referring agency before you meet. Hence, the client is likely to be receptive to seeing you. Even suspicious persons may respond positively, though tentatively. And you must be prepared to meet a variety of clients.

Yet a positive reception cannot be assured. The referral process itself may be flawed. For example, the client may see the referral as punishment for unacceptable behavior, or as a process to compensate for her personal deficits. Or she may see you as a poor substitute for a professional. Further, it may be something as simple as a poorly timed referral. For any of these reasons, the client may be reluctant to participate in visiting, and may reject help altogether, especially if she is suspicious and/or feels the relationship will be too demanding. In such circumstances you must tread lightly, listen and reassure the client. It is difficult to know the client's immediate disposition, so a positive and gentle contact may compensate for an otherwise poor beginning. If the effort breaks down, plan to do the necessary repair work and try again, perhaps a week later.

Caregivers and Setting Must Be Observed

In addition to helping the client, you must talk with the caregivers, assuming she has such, and read the client's chart if such is maintained, to keep fully abreast of the client's condition and program. What do the caregivers say about her condition and participation in activities? Are the caregivers attentive, concerned, constructive, and knowledgeable about the client and committed to her care?

Also, the residence must be observed. Is it clean? Does it have an odor? Is it dismal or cheerfully decorated? Is it comfortably furnished, lighted, heated, and does it have the necessary safeguards to protect the client from accidents?

Goals and Objectives

As sweeping as it sounds, the goal of monitoring and working with elderly persons includes protecting and enhancing their quality of life. Though achievable, candor requires noting that this goal is qualified by the condition of the client, including her physical and mental health, and by her family situation. These conditions may often be poor and the prognosis guarded. While the limitations are often substantial, you can make an appreciable difference in the client's outlook, morale and sense of well being in many cases.

The problems and potentials of the elderly person and her circumstances influence the choice of intervention goals. These goals may be broad, such as enhancing the client's quality of life, or may be specific, to help the client cope with an emergency such as panic about dying, suicidal preoccupation, upset over family relationships or serious dissatisfaction over the quality of care. Specific objectives seek the client's return to her pre-crisis level of getting along. The broader goal seeks not only to improve her daily life but to help her resolve personal problems, including ones from the past.

The psychological part of work with the elderly develops as the person brings various aspects of her life into the conversation. Though her worries will not likely be presented in a systematic or orderly way, they eventually make up a pattern of causal factors and consequences in the course of her dialogue. Aspects of early childhood influence the experience of adolescence, and they in turn contribute to the early, middle and late stages of adulthood. The experiences of each of these phases of life—the good/bad, the constructive/destructive—relate to what happens next until the life course is complete.

The influences of parents, siblings, peers, teachers and others in authority interact with the maturational drives of the individual, and contribute to the child's and adolescent's personality— disposition, adjustment, and point of view. As the person moves forward through adulthood and to later life, her personality retains many of these characteristics (and unresolved personal problems), though the person will obviously be a different or modified person in old age from her earlier years because of the intervening experiences and biological changes. With the cumulative effect of losses typically experienced in older years, there is also the prospect of the person turning more inward in later life.

The objectives of monitoring are specific in contrast to those with visiting in the interest of the elderly person's psychological and social needs. The monitoring includes:

(1) checking the client's care, noting any relevant changes as indicated by her appearance, comments or complaints; (2) reporting perceived changes to the person(s) in charge, for example, a family member or guardian, a social worker or charge nurse; and (3) giving incidental and

concrete service, such as accompanying her to the hospital, purchasing clothes and contacting a relative or friend.

Once goals and a general way of proceeding have been set, just what to do, and when, are the commanding questions. Yet confident answers are often not always available. Factors to consider include the physical and psychosocial status of the client, her particular mood and intellectual predilections at the moment, your own skill and the family and social circumstances. Considerations of specific approaches and techniques follow later.

II
Candidates For Volunteer Attention

The Clients

Candidates for volunteer attention include a broad range of elderly, especially those who are lonesome, isolated, afflicted with poor physical health or mental illness, or both, and whose family ties and contact with friends are limited, if existent at all. Some such persons are likely to have a sponsor—a friend, family, guardian or social worker—who will contact you for assistance. If the contact is made by a professional, the needs and expectations are likely to be clear; however, if a lesser skilled person makes the contact, you may need to explore the details of the case carefully before making a commitment.

This is not to suggest that other elderly persons are not candidates as well. This includes those who are still engaged with family and friends, in modestly good health and fully ambulatory, and who may seek help on their own because of some psychological stress; or those who desire help in planning their care, immediate or future; or who are interested in a close relationship with an understanding, supportive person.

However, humaneness calls for priority attention to be given to those in greatest need—the elderly who lack the necessary physical or mental capacity to make fully appropriate decisions about their daily life and care. They may live in their own homes, perhaps helped by a nursing assistant, or in a group home, or in a nursing home. They may be under guardianship because of their lost capacities. They will be referred to alleviate loneliness, despondency or depression. In some instances, the person may be agitated, even combative. Others may be out of contact with reality, or largely so. Still others may be losing their sense of person and speech because of a mental illness.

You may see a debilitated case to monitor her care and work with her caregivers to ensure quality care. As suggested earlier, in such a circumstance you are likely to have a supportive relationship to the elderly person.

With the more intact, expressive clients, you will seek to actively engage the person interpersonally through interviewing. This interchange encourages the client to express her interests, activities, relationships and feelings in the present and past as you help her review and understand them.

More in Regard to the Client

There are great variations in people over age 65 in such areas as physical status, vitality, personality adjustment, religious and moral values, personal nuances and eccentricities, social and economic class characteristics, access to health care and other services and relatedness to family and friends.

With aging, there is a gradual slowing down in the division, growth, and repair of cells. Consequently, the elderly person typically functions at a less efficient level and has decreased recuperative ability after injury or disease. The body's balance is less efficient among its neuromuscular system, cardiac system and endocrine glands, all of which maintain the person's basic physiological functions such as temperature, respiratory rate, blood volume and pressure, and oxygen supply to the tissues. Also, the central nervous system degenerates and results in slowed reaction time to stimuli, decreased learning capacity, impaired memory and intellectual functioning, and distortions about time, place and person. Associated with these degenerative changes are an uncertain gait, impaired ability to balance the body, loss of hearing, and a variety of diseases, including chronic brain syndromes. In the psychological sphere, the body's reduced capacity to produce energy is likely to be associated with lower sexual energy or libido, less active outreach to others and reduced work capacity. Increased passive needs, self-interest and concern, as well as self-preservation, are also likely to be expressed. These characteristics are shown differently among the elderly, and it is unlikely that any person will manifest all of them.

Mental Problems

Mental problems stem from a number of illnesses, psychological, neurological and physical. Among the psychological are anxiety, fear and panic, paranoia, depressions, overly aggressive behavior, inappropriate sexual behavior, and alcohol and drug abuse. The neurological illnesses include Alzheimer's, a type of senile dementia, strokes, and Parkinson's disease. Other illnesses such as cancer, diabetes, and arthritis are likely to cause the person mental problems.

Socially, the network of friends shrinks for the elderly, especially as they lose formerly held social roles, such as those of an employee, professional, church officer or active member, spouse, neighbor or community leader. As a result, they are more likely to be isolated, lonely and restricted to less than adequate social activity. Social and cultural differences among the elderly, especially as these differences pertain to language, economic level, customs and traditions, must be given your special attention, as they may be problematic for the client. A referral to a mental health professional is recommended if the client's situation is acute in any of the conditions described below. This does not mean you should stop seeing the client. Instead, seek the counsel of the professional for techniques and style of relating to the client, and continue to contribute in the way that is worked out with the professional. Generally, an at-ease, matter-of-fact, unhurried style should help calm the elderly person. That, combined with active listening, perhaps over a lengthy period, will ease the person's agitation.

Anxiety, Fear and Panic may be associated with other illnesses, immediate disturbing circumstances, dismal future prospects or unresolved personal problems stemming from earlier traumatic events. But whatever the cause, the person is distressed and exceedingly uncomfortable. Her ability to concentrate, attend and follow through to action is impaired.

Depressions may range from downheartedness to deep despair. Persons experiencing a mild to moderate depression may be quiet, restrained, inhibited, discouraged, self-deprecating and may have a pervasive feeling of weariness, inadequacy and hopelessness. They probably have difficulty making decisions or may be completely unable to do so. Not only are they likely to feel overly burdened and preoccupied with personal problems, their thinking is slackened. Chronic complaining about physical ailments for which no medical support can be found, loss of concentration, increased anxiety and sleep disturbances may be a part of this condition.

Persons experiencing more intense depressions are gripped by deep despondency and guilt. They are self-accusatory, overwhelmed with personal agonies and are difficult to engage in conversation. Further, they may be highly tense, anxious, confused, feel their surroundings are unreal and be at risk for suicide.

Paranoia, which may be part of a schizophrenia, is expressed by unrealistic wariness, suspicion and accusations of others. Though her suspicions are unjust and untrue, the person is convinced of them and acts on them. Other symptoms include irrational anger, agitation and delusions. It is key that you not become entangled in the paranoid person's suspicions and delusions. You must be objective, matter-of-fact and empathic but not overly involved.

Overly Aggressive Behavior may accompany the paranoid person's agitated, wary behavior. However, this behavior is also related to frustrations and disappointments. The care staff are the most likely targets for attacks; you may be lashed out at too. Avoid stimulating the client's aggression. Instead, a calm, soft-spoken, empathic approach is likely to have a calming effect.

Inappropriate Sexual Behavior stems from sexual impulses continuing into old age without appropriate outlets and failing social awareness and inhibitions. So the person may make untoward advances toward others, or masturbate in the presence of others or expose himself to others.

Remaining calm and encouraging others to do the same is essential, as such situations are likely to generate high-pitched emotions and concerns about morality and etiquette. Discreet handling of a sexual episode, nursing home policy considerations and face-to-face consultation with the elderly person may help the situation. Denial, evasiveness, and down-playing of the episode by the elderly person may be expected.

Alcoholism and Drug Abuse, including the overuse of prescription and over-the-counter drugs, is a problem with some elderly. If the person is in a nursing home, the problem is likely to be under control. It is less likely to be controlled in a group home, or in assisted living; there is less supervision there. The greatest possibility for an elderly person to engage in some form of addiction is when living independently.

In any of these addictive situations, the problem is likely to be denied by the elderly person and often by those about her, including the family. The excessive drinking or pill-taking may be routine, that is, daily, or it may be periodic and related to stress. Anxiety often lies behind the addicted person's denial, and complicates the matter. A confrontation, done matter-of-factly, and referral to a professional should be done. A report to your supervisor is essential.

In the realm of addiction is the possibility that the nursing home encourages the overuse of prescription drugs out of ignorance, or deliberately to control disruptive behavior.

Alzheimer's Disease, a type of senile dementia, though usually slow and gradual in its development, is irreversible. Several typical symptoms are memory loss, personality change, agitation and anxiety, sleeplessness and wandering, failure to recognize immediate family members, disorientation to time and space and failure to know oneself. These symptoms become more severe as the disease advances. Yet there may be moments when the person's memory may flicker back to its earlier capacity, and the recognition of persons and places with it.

During the early phase of the disease let her lead the way on what she wants to talk about. As the disease progresses your major contribution is to the care staff. In that realm, you should support their arranging the most comfortable and secure setting for the client.

Small Strokes produce dizziness, mild weakness of a leg or arm, or slurred speech, but do not result in a major paralysis or loss of speech. On the other hand, severe strokes cause paralysis on one side of the body. Yet in some instances there is no paralysis, or if so, only temporary.

Further, some persons have their speech affected, as well as their capacity to understand language. Also, the ability to read, write, and/or make good judgments may be lost. It depends on which part of the brain was damaged by bleeding from a ruptured blood vessel.

Parkinson's Disease is a progressive neurological disorder. Persons having it will be shaky and have difficulty in making simple movements such as walking or handling objects. Their speech may be affected and their facial expressions are absent. Chewing and swallowing may also be affected. All of these symptoms are caused by muscle rigidity. Depression and discouragement are often associated with the illness.

You may help the client and family members cope with the exceptional stress of the illness by offering support, realistic encouragement and empathy. It is important for you to be there for them.

III

Practical Considerations and Initial Moves

Time and Space

To develop and sustain a working relationship with an elderly client, you should see her at least once a week. Such time is necessary to make meaningful contact, develop a continuity of presence, establish a mode of communication and generate a bond of sentiment. It also helps construct trust and dependability and encourages the client to express her concerns and relate them from one visit to another.

You should spend considerable time with the client, about forty minutes per visit. Short visits are very unlikely to generate or sustain a working relationship, even if they are pleasant. Whatever length of time is agreed upon, you must limit the visit to that, even though the client may attempt various maneuvers to continue when the time to close is reached. The elderly person may withhold significant items to the end of the meeting to extend the time. On the other hand, the client may seek to end an interview early to escape talking about an anxiety-loaded problem. So you must be aware.

You must not opt out of a session because it is unproductive, even dull. Though tedious, waiting and working through these periods are often necessary to pursue relevant concerns.

The time with the client should not be interrupted, which may be difficult to maintain in a group or nursing home with its many routines and procedures. If interruptions occur more than occasionally, the matter should be discussed with the charge nurse to work out a time and place where the interviews can be sustained. Privacy increases the likelihood of the client's sharing her inner thoughts. Further, it is important that both the client and you are seated comfortably, and that your chairs are on the same level.

If the client is in her home and benefitting from the care of an in-home nursing assistant or family member, you may need to involve them in some

15

parts of the interviews, especially if the client has difficulty verbalizing or if the client's care is under discussion. Generally, however, the time should be for the elderly person alone.

Starting the Interviewing

Interviewing begins with the first visit. After a friendly greeting and casual conversation, you should informally outline the prospects of a relationship. Speaking informally, conversational style, you must tell the elderly person the major parts of the anticipated relationship. It's best if you can weave it into your conversation. However, it may be appropriate to spell it out immediately, particularly if the client is receptive. For example, speaking easily, you might say, "I've come because I'm interested in the welfare of senior citizens and you were recommended by your agency. My responsibility is to visit regularly—once a week for forty minutes, listen to you, ask about your joys and worries, and occasionally comment. Your part is to take time to see me, and to talk about what is important to you. The purpose is to make you more comfortable, feel better. You, of course, are free to drop out at any time."

    You must be certain to draw the elderly person into the conversation, particularly to have her ask questions about the basic character of the relationship and about the nature of future visits. In this process, you and the client will address the point of whether the elderly person wants to engage in such a relationship, what her responsibilities will be, as well as what yours will be. Along with addressing these questions, you must encourage the elderly person to express any hesitancies that she may have. It is often helpful to suggest that she postpone her decision about developing a visiting relationship until the next visit, after she has had a week to think it over. The elderly person must have the right to refuse to see you, even if she is under guardianship and needs the social support and psychological help being offered.

    Further, you must explain your presence to the facility staff and other relevant persons, if this has not been previously done. They are responsible for the client, are concerned about her and may seriously wonder, but not express to you, the question of what you can add to what they are already doing. A friendly, matter-of-fact approach should convey your interest. Neither an apologetic nor a demanding introduction is appropriate. Instead, an "easy" entree should do it. Among your requests are opportunities to read the client's chart and subsequently contribute to it, talk to the elderly person in private and assure the confidentiality of your talks with the client.

As suggested earlier, you should present the opportunity for a helping relationship during the first call and let her decide at the second visit, a week later, whether she wants to continue. If the client is lucid or even modestly so, the style of these early visits should be clear, to the point and friendly. The emphasis of these visits is to get the client to talk and express herself on whatever topics she chooses. It is not to be a forum for you to talk. Instead, you must listen patiently and ask questions occasionally to help the client clarify herself, detail what she has in mind, tie emotions and related ideas together, explore ideas and earlier experiences and tie them to her current thinking.

The client may ask about your motivations and about your background. Short, candid answers are appropriate, all given without defensive explanation. You should not over-explain yourself. Indeed, to do so will probably make the elderly person uneasy. Moreover, it is not an occasion to display your resume.

The elderly person may make exploratory ventures in response to your proposal by expressing dissatisfaction with her current living situation, the condition of her health or an earlier life experience. You must listen closely, help her elaborate and develop the details of her concern and generally help her get started. This is the pattern that should be established. There may be some matters on which you can be of direct help, such as talking with the care staff about aspects of the client's care or the activities of her program.

If the client has a poor memory, or is somewhat confused or shy, you must take the initiative. You may have to repeat, help the elderly person over critical moments, be patient and be certain to reassure. Brain damage may retard the client, or she may be afraid or distrustful. Hence you might introduce something that is immediate to her experience—an activity she has engaged in, or the menu of a lunch just completed or the decorations of the residence. All such efforts aim to get the elderly person to talk.

Once the elderly person has "tested the waters" by introducing an item of conversation, she will have gotten the acquaintance underway. You may need to make some queries to continue the process. If the client is highly recalcitrant, or shy, or handicapped in her speech, you will have to be patient and gently persist in getting a session started. Typically, the elderly person's chosen topic, either deliberately chosen or fortuitously arrived at, has excellent prospects for development, and even if only incidental, it may serve as a jumping-off point to related areas of importance. The client may be encouraged to elaborate her initial remarks, or move to associated topics by making favorable comment and asking pertinent but unobtrusive questions. With such stimulation the conversation should move ahead.

Before ending the second session, you must be sure the elderly person understands the possibility of developing an extended relationship, and finally, you should shake the elderly person's hand, thereby affirming your interest, and say one or a number of positive things before leaving. If the client has expressed an interest in continuing, you should enter the time and date of her next appointment on her calendar, or encourage her to do it.

The second visit may even be more important than the first one. As suggested earlier, the client's expectations and hopes of a continuing relationship may include being befriended, encouraged, guided and advised, all to improve her morale. However, the client may feel differently, and may not want to be encumbered by someone whom she does not know and feels may be too demanding or too nosy. Or, if her speech is impaired because of a stroke or dementia, she may reject visits because she is agitated or feels unable to speak well enough. The uncertainties of completing a helping arrangement include other possibilities. For example, the elderly person may have forgotten the details of the first visit, and even you. Whatever the circumstances, you must talk with the client early on during the second meeting about whether she wants to continue.

These several variations in response, and there are others, not only reflect personality differences among clients but also indicate their variations in health, mental health, and social circumstances.

Obtaining Information

As the elderly person has gained in years, not only has she acquired some of the typical problems of the elderly — for example, loss of energy, diminished sight, hearing, taste, smell, locomotion and so on — but she also is likely to have acquired a disease of one kind or another—often more than one. Further, the elderly person will have acquired a history, a record, by virtue of her trips to doctors' and social workers' offices, hospitals, health and social agencies, and, if she is under guardianship, to the court.

The circumstances associated with your initial contact will vary. It will be especially helpful if you have read the client's history as well as having been briefed by the referring person.

Once contact has been made with the elderly person, you will have opportunities to make observations and ask appropriately sensitive questions to understand the elderly person and her situation concretely and to fully assess the current situation and the history for yourself.

The Elderly Person's Behavior During the Visit

What the elderly person says, the way she says it, with special gestures, tone of voice and emphasis, should indicate what preoccupies her and how she feels about it. Though probably not complete or detailed, her statements may say something about the causes of her preoccupation.

Several things are typically covered, or conveyed in what she says and how she says it. First, there is the substance of the elderly person's concern — for example, the lack of activity in the nursing home, the estrangement from children, the pain associated with illness. Second is the emotion attached to the concern — for example, her anxiety, disappointment, despair or anger. Third is the manner in which she handles her concern and anger, as by taking some type of direct action or by wringing her hands and doing nothing. Fourth are the factors causing her preoccupation, such as the progressive course of an illness, an unresolved family quarrel, or an unresolved loss of a spouse through death.

Again, the range in what the elderly person may do varies. Not all statements will have substantive material that allows the aforementioned analysis. For example, to guard against making a self-deprecating comment, the client may initially say something to enhance her person, even though it may be exaggeration. However, the responses are varied, as has been suggested, and the elderly person, driven by a poor sense of personal worth and depression, may deprecate herself or remain passive and say nothing. The possibilities are substantial, as she may be very talkative but be confused and offer distortions and fabrications, or she may chatter about irrelevant matters to stay away from important issues.

Associated with any of the problems that have been mentioned is the prospect of the client crying. Your safest reaction is to permit and perhaps encourage the client to cry if such is on the surface—to get it out. Once it is out, the client may be somewhat relieved and you can help her consider the matter of concern. Support and empathy are absolute ingredients in this endeavor.

The Volunteer's Behavior During the Visit

A number of suggestions have already been made about your approach. A list follows, with some repetition. The order does not imply priority of importance, nor does it suggest any sequence for application in the process of working with the elderly. Also, the list does not claim to be all-inclusive. Consistent application of these suggestions, however, should advance your work.

- Be prepared to work with a broad range of clients.
- Show respect, politeness, concern, empathy, and confidence to the client.
- Generate trust in the relationship.
- Be affirming without being sticky-sweet.
- Be dependable, consistent and accountable.
- Be observing of the client and her care.
- Invite the client to express herself, and be a listener.
- Know what is being conveyed and what is not.
- Be a thinker about the client. What is she about? How can she be helped? Be a student of your work.
- Give attention to the client's immediate concern even though it seems clear that it has powerful underlying roots. Attend to first things first. Provide some psychological relief through empathy and support. Once such relief is provided, you may help the client bring underlying and associated factors to the fore.
- Be a good reporter to the persons who ultimately are responsible for the client—a family member or spouse, or guardian— particularly at points of crisis.
- Always be mindful that information about the client is confidential and is not to be shared with the public, even with your closest friends. If compelled to share a scenario, do not use names or other identifying characteristics. Rather, speak of the individual's condition, and the action being taken to help it.
- As has already been suggested, closely observe the quality of the client's care. In greater detail: Is she clean, neatly dressed? Is her hair combed? Nails done? Does she have any unexplained, or even explained, bruises? Does the facility or the client have an odor? Particularly, if she lives independently, is she eating regularly and what is the make-up of her diet? Also, in addition to observing, ask the client matter-of-factly about the quality of her care and her degree of satisfaction.

Continuing the Clinical Arrangement

Assuming the client has agreed to be visited, you may anticipate your third meeting with the client somewhat in the character of the earlier efforts. If the client was quiet and uncommunicative, she is apt to continue that style. Or if the client was talkative, she will continue in that manner. Whatever the client's response, you must further the rapport, the relationship, the communication. If the client has been quiet, and you believe she has the mental capacity to share her experience and views, you must spend some time sitting in silence, as the client may seek to wait you out, that is, for you to do the talking while she takes a passive and waiting role. You are advised to move carefully, explore the situation, sympathize, encourage, empathize, and not to conjecture or offer interpretations. You should not be discouraged, but remember that the process is in its very early phase and many opportunities to engage the client will follow.

On the other hand, if the client talked in the earlier sessions, she can be expected to continue. She may knowingly or unknowingly display her hopes, fears and wishes, yet guard her painful past memories and even distress over her current condition. However, all these are likely to be expressed at a later time.

The earlier the main aspects of the client's concerns can be grasped, the better. Some of that can be gained from studying the client's record, but it still must be seen and played out in the visits. Experiences expressed in interviews have an immediate reality. This is different from a historical recording and allows you to explore, and the client to bring her concerns into the open.

Working with Care Staff

As has been suggested earlier, if the client is in a group or nursing home, or in an assisted living residence, you should consult with the care staff—charge nurse, nursing assistants, physical therapists, recreational personnel—to learn of the client's condition, whether any progress is being made, and if you may be of any assistance.

It is well for you to appreciate the stress under which these people work and their need for support, encouragement and recognition. So you must provide reassurance and any technical help you are able to give, and thank them for monitoring information.

In some instances the relationship between you and the care staff will be different. For example, when the client is a custodial case, or near to it, and cannot communicate actively, you may spend a short period with the client to attempt to communicate, to exchange some feelings, and to monitor her condition. The remainder of your time may be invested in conferring with and supporting the care staff's daily efforts.

For example, they may be exasperated by the behavior of an Alzheimer's patient, her wandering, sleeplessness and nighttime disturbances, packing and unpacking her belongings, her loss of self-identity and speech, and her incontinence. This may be complicated by the staff's coping with the death and dying of other persons. Whether the staff is new to the work or highly experienced, listening and supporting them will help.

The Volunteer's Supervision and Liaison

In all likelihood your work will be under someone's supervision— typically a social worker or psychologist—a person who is trained and experienced in working with the elderly. The supervisor, as well as the client, is likely to be affiliated with an agency, particularly if the client is under guardianship. The supervisor can help you in several ways: screening and referring clients, advising on client dynamics and your technique, evaluating the progress of the case and working with family members and others who may be legally involved in the case.

As you begin to feel at ease with your supervisor, you may want to share your personal reactions to clients, including your negative and upset feelings, all of which can be worked through for your comfort and improvement, and to the benefit of the client.

Loss as a Serious Concern

Aged persons will usually have suffered painful losses in their lives, deaths of others especially. Their parents, significant relatives, and perhaps siblings will have died, and though these deaths may have been years in the past, the images and feelings may have continued. Without the grief having been resolved, the aged person mourns for these persons in the present—not always openly, but privately.

Death of the client's children, as infants or as adults, also may be sources of painful memories and sadness for the elderly person. Probably pressed by life's many demands at the time of such deaths, the aged person did not grieve for them sufficiently to get some closure on these traumas. Now, in old age, the person's grief continues as an unresolved problem.

Typically, the most serious loss in old age is the death of a spouse. Even if it happened several years previously, the hurt may still be very current and unresolved.

Loss as a serious problem also includes those caused by personal ill health: the loss of eyesight and hearing, the loss of locomotion (walking, standing, etc.), the loss of friends and family, the loss of money and economic security. These losses are not only devastating by their direct impact, but by their negative effect on the client's sense of identity, independence, personal worth, pride and hope. Giving the client an opportunity to ventilate her feelings and giving her support should help.

Nonverbal Communication

Elderly people, as others, shrug their shoulders, close their eyes, raise their eyebrows, shake or nod their heads, smile or laugh, sit rigidly or constantly turn in their chairs, frown, grimace, become tearful, extend their arms, open and close their hands, and so on as ways of communicating without speaking. These nuances are often called body language. In addition, there are cues the client gives about her feelings by tone of voice, whether it is highly pitched, or soft and hardly audible, or very loud and threatening.

You may respond to these non-stated communications intuitively—that is, naturally—without giving them a second thought. Further, you may have unique ways of communicating without talking or even uttering a sound. It is important for you to be aware of your own manner of communicating, as well as that of the client, to be sure of the full meaning of your conversation.

Feelings are Important

Given the importance of feelings—happiness, sadness, anger, fear and so on—you must be especially sensitive to them. Often the positive ones are expressed openly or are close to the surface and can be easily tapped. Happy ones associated with enjoyable past experiences add to the client's morale and sense of well being. The negative feelings—sadness, anger, fear—are more complex because they may not be reached easily, and, when expressed, may disturb the client. So why not leave them alone? Because they are burdensome to the elderly person and if called forth gently by you and worked through, she will be relieved of them.

These ventures should not be attempted until you have a close relationship with the client, and they must be done carefully and progressively, not by your jumping in with abandon.

Intense Problems

The client may revolt against her living situation, or cry out from excruciating pain, or remain mute in a deep depression, threaten suicide in desperation or cry, fearing death. These and related dramatic matters call for immediate action, and they are usually met by a physician, psychiatrist, nurse, social worker or nursing assistant, or perhaps a family member, leaving you in a support position. Yet that role may be crucial, especially in giving support to the client or care staff or direct service to the client.

Also, by following a case closely, you may see a problem building to dangerous proportions and de-escalate it, and/or call for the assistance of others. Moreover, you should join with others to review the problem after it has been handled to see how it came about and learn whether it might have been foreseen in advance.

Mental Medications

The client with a mental problem will often be on medication. The various medications, the conditions they are used for and the effects they are likely to have are described in Appendix B. Other information is given there, including possible side effects and precautions.

IV

General Approaches and Techniques

The manner of relating to the elderly is broken into two parts:1) general approaches, and 2) techniques. The *general approaches* are your basic ways of positioning yourself to the elderly person, your main attitudes or dispositions. They include being self-aware, courageous, kind, friendly, trustworthy and perceptive.

What you do specifically are *techniques*, such as observation; empathy and taking the role of the elderly person; affirmation and support; active listening; encouraging expression; talking-sharing and suggesting; persisting; teaching; normalizing; reviewing, clarifying and focusing; and summarizing.

This organization of ways to relate to the elderly has overlaps in the different methods, and could include additional items. But it will get you underway and help you in your work.

General Approaches

Self Awareness

Self awareness is important in working with the elderly. Specifically, you need to be aware of how you typically perceive ("size up") situations and persons, how you act and react to them, especially those who have problems, and how you affect others.

Such self-awareness enhances not only your understanding of yourself, but also the reactions of the client, all of which aim to make you more helpful.

Example: Mrs. I. T.

Mrs. I. T., a former teacher and widow, was at the nursing home due to a stroke which partially paralyzed her. A wheelchair gave her mobility and she used it occasionally to go to activities and visit other patients. She was a quiet woman, very quiet, and worn down. She saw the volunteer because she was downcast. Though usually conversive, she was reluctant to talk on this particular day. She led with an item, then dropped it and rejected the volunteer's efforts to have her continue. Hoping to have Mrs. I. T. continue, and momentarily unmindful of the rule to keep his personal experiences out of his work, the volunteer spoke about his relationship to a sister. "I know just what you must mean. Things don't always go well, or the way you want them to go. On one occasion . . ." Then he caught himself, became aware that he was foisting a unique experience onto the client, and shifted. "You've mentioned your sister several times, but you haven't really developed the matter."

Example: Mrs. Q.

The volunteer's schedule at the nursing home typically brought him to Mrs. Q.'s geri chair about 11:00 a.m. The nursing home began serving its noon lunch shortly after that. With him present, however, the nursing assistants skipped Mrs. Q., planning to serve her after the volunteer left. Mrs. Q., however, was used to eating on schedule. She fidgeted and stopped talking as she saw trays being served to other clients. Then the volunteer grasped the situation, begged her pardon, and asked the nursing assistants to serve Mrs. Q. They did, and the visiting continued.

Friendship

Friendship involves you, as a volunteer, extending yourself to the client in an amicable, congenial, sociable, warmhearted manner. Initially this is done to get acquainted, but in the longer term, it aims at bonding with her in a close, harmonious way. It is well meant and generous. The warmth of the relationship is shown by time, talk and understanding to assist the elderly person in her isolation and despair, and affirms her person. Friendship is a comfortable, unpretending, and candid relationship that mixes hope, desire, optimism and faith with realistic appraisals of serious matters, including death and dying. It rests on trust, confidence, kindness, benevolence, accord, compatibility, assurance and the emotions of happiness and despair. It is a relationship in which you must be a supporter, upholder and advocate for the elderly person.

Friendship is the keystone to all techniques and approaches.

Example: Mr. Z.

Mr. Z. was an eighty-two-year-old former teacher and widower, who was plagued by cancer of the pancreas. The volunteer saw him at a nursing home once a week for an hour over a period of four months. He was a tall, thin intellectual who enjoyed talking about meteorology, his profession. The volunteer encouraged, supported and listened to his reminiscing. Together, they got along well.

In addition, politics, economics and social problems, religious interests, health, ill health, medical care and current events were discussed, put aside unresolved, but resurfaced again and again.

Mr. Z. became more and more infirm as the cancer progressed but did his best to sit up in an easy chair for the visits, and the conversation took on a heavy air as Mr. Z. talked about his imminent death. A common bond of friendship, a reciprocity of positive feelings in each other developed early and was strengthened throughout the four months; and as the end was imminent, the feelings were sustained. At first Mr. Z.'s concern was shrouded in desperation and fear. Then it turned philosophical. "It has to end sometime." As his pain increased, he sought death as a relief. Every trace of color was drained out of his once-ruddy face, leaving him dull and opaque as clay. His wide, grey eyes stared hard and intense like steel. For long moments he sat or lay in bed without moving or saying a word. His grey lips were drawn in pain and sometimes cast in a bitter smile.

Clearly aware of what was taking place, the volunteer braced himself for the death that would soon take his friend. And it did, the day of his last regular visit. The client lay in bed with his eyes closed and responded only with a slight nod of his head as the volunteer held his hand.

The volunteer left the group home and stopped at the gate leading onto the street. He stood there. His hand reached down to turn the latch. Somehow he missed it and instead grasped the post immediate to the latch. He gripped it, both for support and to release tension. After a moment he loosened his grip, unlatched the gate and walked to his car, and as he opened the door, tears ran down his cheeks.

Example: Mr. Y.

Mr. Y. was a seventy-nine-year-old stroke victim and widower whom the volunteer listened to, empathized with, supported, and encouraged. These interactions generated a distinct relationship of mutual respect and good will—a friendship. With sandy, graying hair trimmed short, and small, shrewd, alert features, Mr. Y. was always ready to engage in a give-and-take conversation.

Conversation took place in an atmosphere of mutual confidence, spontaneity, openness, and ease. The volunteer asked Mr. Y. about his earlier life and education. Mr. Y. asked the volunteer to share his. The volunteer asked Mr. Y. about his career and the volunteer reciprocated to Mr. Y.'s inquiry. Current affairs and politics were discussed and different views were exchanged. The close of each session was typically concluded by each thanking the other for his time and expressing his anticipations for the next meeting.

Courage

Courage refers to persisting with the elderly in spite of their rejection, lukewarm acceptance or indifference, confused verbalization, anxiety attacks, depression, progressive illness, demise and dying.

Working with the elderly includes more positive experiences than the ones indicated above. The positive experiences and the challenges of working through the negative ones contribute greatly to your sustenance as a volunteer. However, the sustenance also comes from your basic courage to face human crisis—indeed, the critical matter of life and death.

Example: Mr. B.

Mr. B. was a seventy-nine-year-old terminal cancer patient whom the volunteer initially visited weekly at a group home to monitor his care. He was a widower with no immediate family. The monitoring turned to friendship as the contact continued; however, Mr. B.'s health deteriorated as his cancer progressed. His vision failed, pain ravished his body, his ankles swelled and his strength lapsed until he was no longer able to walk. His once-vivid recollections of a happy childhood, stimulating college life, and successful scientific career were lost. He fell attempting to walk and was transferred from his group home to a hospital, where his condition "stabilized." He was moved to a nursing home. There his condition worsened. The volunteer continued to see him, but Mr. B. discontinued reflecting about his past and was quiet most of the time, excepting when he complained, ever so quietly, about his excruciating pain.

The volunteer listened, supported, and empathized as Mr. B. contemplated his death. At the same time the volunteer struggled with his sadness about Mr. B.'s imminent passing. It was courage, more than knowledge of the life cycle, that sustained him.

Mr. B. died, a day after the volunteer last saw him. The volunteer was shaken out of his normal calm. He had unwittingly hoped that somehow or other Mr. B. would live just a while longer. That, however, was not to be, and when the volunteer learned of Mr. B.'s death, he stood quietly for some time, stricken by grief, and then turned to do immediately pressing work, and later in the day some physical activity.

The effect of working with the elderly may impinge on the volunteer's unconscious, as is shown in the following dream.

That night as the volunteer slept, he dreamt that he called on Mr. B. and sat by his side in the group home as he had done dozens of times. Mr. B. smiled softly as they conversed, nodded his head easily, and looked down at the floor. In his dream, the volunteer suspected that Mr. B. was dead. Yet he was not sure, and he felt he must be especially sensitive or Mr. B. would fade away and be gone forever. Considerable tension followed as the volunteer tried to converse with Mr. B. He did not answer but smiled, nodded his head and looked at the floor. He didn't seem unhappy and was not in pain, but he did not respond. The tension awoke the volunteer and he realized that he had been dreaming. He lay looking up at the ceiling of the bedroom, downhearted, yet he knew that his relationship to Mr. B. had been a fine one.

Example: Mrs. O.

Mrs. O., an eighty-seven-year-old, non-complaining yet sensitive widow, was receiving chemotherapy for cancer at a nursing home. The chemotherapy had the adverse effect of clouding her vision. "First it was my left eye, then my right one, now both." She rose unsteadily and pulled a piece of paper from a stack of books on her side table. "Here, look at this," she said as she extended the medical prescription to the volunteer. Her voice was uncertain, and the anxiety was clear. "You know, I never noticed this before. Guess I couldn't see it, or read it, but right here it says the possible side effects, and sure enough, it says 'impaired vision may occur'."

She watched the volunteer for his reaction, hoping for support. Her teeth were clenched and her jaw was set.

Mixing empathy with matter-of-factness, and searching for courage, the volunteer repeated, "Impaired vision may occur."

Mrs. O. responded, "I never bargained for this, don't want it, but I don't have any choice. So I'll do the best I can with it." She nodded her head to affirm her view, but the sadness of her voice was clear as a bell.

The volunteer caught its full impact and reached over to her chair and gently touched her hand and said, "I know. I know."

She grasped his hand tightly. Her courage touched him. Indeed enhanced his courage. He repeated, "I know, I know."

Kindness

While objectivity must be sustained in the client relationship, a generous, benevolent, accommodating, attentive regard must prevail alongside it. Being considerate and obliging—indeed, performing acts of grace—are essential. That disposition will carry you a long way in your work.

Example: Mr. G. A.

Mr. G. A. was a tall, slender man with watery blue eyes and a distinguished gray handlebar mustache. He was outgoing but suffered from lapses of memory. His memory problem made it impossible for him to manage the routines of maintaining his checkbook. Hence, he had a guardian of property. He was widowed, and had no immediate family near or interested in maintaining contact.

A volunteer saw him weekly at a nursing home to maintain his morale and help with his occasional bouts with depression. Though the progress of the visiting was satisfactory, Mr. G. A. moved to a city some distance away to be near an adult daughter.

Several months later, the volunteer was vacationing in that city, and after calling Mr. G. A., went by the group home in which he lived—a drive of about twenty miles through city traffic—to visit him. Mr. G. A. was elated, and the volunteer was as well. A warm exchange took place for the next hour and a half as the volunteer and Mr. G talked about his recent experience and about their past relationship.

Example: Mr. X.

Mr. X. was an eighty-year-old, formerly highly successful businessman. However, advancing years and arthritis hindered his mobility, and his failing memory limited his mental competence.

The manager of the group home in which he lived notified his social worker that Mr. X. needed a new pair of pajamas and several pairs of underwear. She, in turn, asked the volunteer to make the purchases. Though this was not in the agreement of what he would do, the volunteer replied, "Sure, I'll do it this week."

Trustworthiness

Being reliable, dependable, predictable—positively so—steadfast and unfailing in respect to the client are key. She must be able to count on the appointments at the allotted time, and on your procedures, your persisting through time and availability in emergencies. On these matters you must be responsible and incorruptible.

Example: Mrs. C. T.

Mrs. C. T. was a seventy-two-year-old widow, a nursing home resident who had a very strained relationship with her husband, caused by his irresponsibility and deceit. That, in turn, seemed to make her cautious with the volunteer and question his motivation. She doubted that he would see her weekly and expressed that boldly at their second meeting. Her doubts persisted until the third month of their contact.

The weather was bad on that particular day. It was snowing, sleeting, and was bitterly cold. The volunteer, however, drove to the nursing home and was greeted by Mrs. C. T., who had been looking out the window to winter outside. She looked at him with combined surprise and consternation. "I wouldn't have believed that such could happen, you know, a couple of months ago, but you're here in spite of everything."

Example: Mrs. F.

Mrs. F. was a seventy-four-year-old angry widow and nursing home resident who had a troubled relationship with her oldest daughter. Neither acknowledged it readily and acted as if it weren't the reality. About six weeks after the volunteer began to see her, Mrs. F. brought this to the fore, first hesitatingly and then very directly. "I don't care how much she pretends, but that marriage of hers is not good. I told her so before she got into it. . . . That was six or seven years ago, but little good that did." After a brief pause she added, "And that's one thing I never want you to say to her. That is, that I told you this!"

The daughter came to visit Mrs. F. a week later, and the volunteer had an opportunity to visit with her when Mrs. F. went for physical therapy. The conversation focused on Mrs. F.'s stay at the nursing home, not the relationship between her and the daughter.

The following week, Mrs. F. recalled the daughter's visit and said with appreciation, "I wasn't sure what you and she would talk about when I was gone, and for a whole hour. I wasn't sure I could trust you, really I didn't, but I learned from Sheila afterwards that you didn't talk about how she and I get along."

Perception

You must be very aware of and sensitive to the client, being able to analyze her remarks and feelings. Such astuteness helps you determine her current status and any changes that have taken place, and then choose a course of action. Similarly, in regard to the care situation, you will be able to discern the quality of what the client is getting.

Example: Mrs. L. N.

Mrs. L. N. was a seventy-six-year-old stroke victim, a widow and resident of a nursing home. She was very responsive to the inquiries of the volunteer, but the responsiveness was typically vague and overly general. She modified this pattern after several months by making indicative comments, but only after the volunteer had terminated the interview. Her tactic defeated the volunteer and saved her from facing her problems. The volunteer sat back down, looked thoughtfully at Mrs. L. N. and suggested, "What you just reported about your husband is not only important, but probably key. But time is up today. Let's start with it next week."

Example: Mr. T. Y.

Mr. T. Y., a seventy-eight-year-old former accountant, widower, and nursing home resident, prided himself on seeing the bright side of matters, including his personal problems, not complaining, and so on. His emphasis was so strong the volunteer suspected Mr. T. Y. was avoiding some difficulty. After letting Mr. T. Y. finish his point, when he seemed to have "run down," the volunteer asked, "Mr. T. Y., do you have an important matter that you haven't brought out?"

Sadly, Mr. T. Y. responded, "You know, in spite of my best efforts, there wasn't any more I could do for her. Her condition was terminal. I took the best care of her that I could, but that wasn't enough. . . . She died."

Techniques

Observation

As a volunteer you must scrutinize the elderly person's appearance, manner, speech, movement, and attitude. Though unobtrusive, the observation is more of a penetrating study than a cursory review. You may need to break your eyes away from the client occasionally as you check over and take stock of her condition. You need to engage in the same careful examination of the client's surroundings and quality of her care. Such inspections are necessary for monitoring. Similarly, the setting, especially its cleanliness, nursing assistants, recreational personnel and the regularity of health care, must be observed.

Example: Mrs. L.

Mrs. L. was a seventy-three-year-old stroke victim who was maintained at home because of her husband's insistence. She was bedridden and required twenty-four-hour nursing care. Earlier, the husband had let her fall into a deplorable condition, failing to provide the minimal hygienic care and nutrition. After complaints by friends, Mrs. L. was brought under guardianship.

The husband was intact mentally; however, his values and commitment to Mrs. L. were highly suspect. Consequently, the observation of both Mr. and Mrs. L. was very close.

On this particular call the volunteer discovered a new nursing assistant had been brought in, but the reason for the previous one's leaving had not been learned. Mr. L. was not at home when the volunteer appeared for the visit. That allowed open conversation with the new nursing assistant. She reported that Mr. L. had been cooperative and that Mrs. L.'s poor condition was unchanged.

Upon returning, Mr. L. arrogantly announced that his priority was to telephone his stockbroker. Though miffed by Mr. L.'s behavior, the volunteer now had a first-hand view of his untoward behavior and an excellent opportunity to speak with Mrs. L. and observe her condition. When this was completed, he left the bedroom for the living room, next to the office in which Mr. L. was conducting his business. Hearing the volunteer prompted Mr. L. to close his telephone conversation and join him. Surprisingly, his earlier arrogance dissolved as he launched into a long story, throwing positive light on his failure to properly care for his wife. He especially dwelt on his despondency, depression and a feeling of complete hopelessness about her condition.

The volunteer listened to Mr. L.'s tense justification, noted its skew in his favor, and advised him so, gently but firmly. Mr. L.'s dismay turned to crying and he repeated his earlier utter helplessness in caring for his wife. He emphasized that it was temporary and that he was doing better.

The volunteer nodded his head slowly. "I see," he said, then continued, "We will monitor her care very closely. That should insure that all goes well."

Mr. L. nodded his head but did not speak.

Example: Mrs. I.

Mrs. I. was a sturdy, seventy-four-year-old widow. Having been a housewife for all of her adult life made her mindful of the housework required to keep a place neat and tidy. Such was not the case in the group home in which she now lived. Instead, the operator stressed that it was a place that emphasized friendship and relationships. The dirt and grime of the home illustrated his point.

The volunteer shared his values and was insensitive to the home's dirtiness; however, his insensitivity was raised after a public health inspection faulted the home on its housekeeping and heating.

On the volunteer's next visit to Mrs. I., he noticed the place was immaculate and a new space heater was in her room.

Mrs. I. began, "Do you see anything different around here?"

"It's all cleaned up and you have a new heater."

"That's right. Now it's a decent place! It's been sloppy, very sloppy. Everybody likes it better now. It's just a better place. Even smells better."

He picked up Mrs. I.'s cue and later complimented the manager, who was pleased and mentioned several additional planned improvements.

As the volunteer left the home and walked down the sidewalk, his reflections of the visit included: "I may have to modify my values and my powers of observation. I just overlooked the earlier sloppiness."

Empathy and Taking the Part of the Elderly Person

Appreciating the elderly person as an important, unique and valuable human being is basic to working with her. You must know this and feel it as well. To achieve such an orientation, you must put yourself into the shoes of the aged person to sense how she looks at and feels about things.

Achieving empathy and taking the part of the elderly person is a subtle undertaking. It requires constant effort, even if one is committed to doing so. It is easy to be analytical and critical of the client's feelings and behavior. Something more and different is needed.

As a volunteer you must look to yourself. "What would I feel like, think and do if I suffered a double stroke? If I were losing my memory and my general competency? If I were ravaged by cancer or diabetes? If I had lost my eyesight or my hearing?" While your feelings and behavior may not be the same as the client's, your reflections on what they might be are an important exercise to appreciating the plight of the elderly person.

Example: Mrs. G.

The client was a sixty-eight-year-old widow who came to the nursing home because assisted home care was not adequate for her several problems: paralysis of her left arm and leg because of a stroke, dementia, aphasia-like speech problems, and alcoholism.

She failed to adapt to the home and complained constantly about "nothing to do," "nobody cares," and so on. Though dissatisfaction was attached to her complaints, the emotion was mild, particularly in contrast to the seriousness of her verbal statements. All in all, she was an unhappy woman, dissatisfied with her nursing home existence, who often viewed the volunteer with raised eyebrows in silent suspicion.

After listening carefully, and showing concern for several visits, the volunteer extended the initial concern to questioning. "Might you feel more upset than you are letting on? I just get that sense in listening to you."

Her face clouded and she exclaimed, "I'm mad, I'm mad, mad about the whole thing and I don't know what I can do," and then charged, "You don't know what it's like to be in the shape I'm in."

The volunteer acknowledged, "You're right. The best I can do is try to appreciate your situation." A silence of several long moments followed. Then the volunteer attempted, "Given what you have said, I know your frustration. Might you consider talking it out? Or better still, might you act on your complaints? For example, you should get more active and enter into the home's activities."

Mrs. G. pursed her lips, pouted for several moments and then spoke. "Well, I might try, but I'm not sure. Besides I don't like those activities." Then, after a long pause, she tentatively offered, "Maybe I'll try something." The volunteer suggested, "Why not? You don't have anything to lose. So try something, or even a few things, this week, and we can talk it over when I come back next week."

"Well, maybe, but I'm not promising anything."

The volunteer left, thinking that Mrs. G. would not act on her complaints. Rather, she would continue to complain. Hence his technical problem was moving her from the complaining to acting. That included allowing her full opportunity to ventilate her anger, and seeing whether it was tied to some earlier life experiences. And it also included examining the benefits she derived by complaining, and any fears she had of acting.

He attempted these several approaches, and though she seemed more at ease and happier, she did not enter any of the activities. Challenged by this, the volunteer suggested, "I'm coming earlier next week, at nine o'clock, the time the activities start. Select one before I come, and I'll take you there."

Example: Mr. C. C.

Mr. C. C., a seventy-nine-year-old retired Marine Corps colonel, spoke at length about his military career, from recruitment to retirement, through the enlisted ranks to that of an officer, then up the line to colonel. His reports were always laudable. Success followed success. Pride in the Corps was always a major theme.

After weeks of this preoccupation, Mr. C. C. slowed down and in a sad voice reported, "You know, I always wanted to make general. I wanted it in the worst way. And you know, I never really knew, still don't know, why I didn't make it."

The volunteer waited an appropriate time, thinking the colonel would continue, but when he did not, the volunteer respectfully suggested, "Might you consider talking about that? I feel it is very important to you."

Affirmation and Support

Affirmation and support mean asserting the client's personal worth, aiming to build her self-esteem. Such is achieved by your presence, the very fact that you come regularly and punctually, convey a positive, friendly yet serious attitude, declare or profess the client's worth and esteem, and assure the elderly person that she can do various achievable tasks. These things convey confidence, understanding and hope to the client.

Along with supporting and sustaining the person, these efforts reinforce or buttress the client's efforts to participate in the interviews—for example, trying to recall life events when she might rather rest.

Example: Mrs. E.

The visitor was about fifty minutes late for his appointment with Mrs. E., a sixty-four-year-old widow with advanced cancer and low self-esteem. After his apology Mrs. E. rasped, "I didn't think you were coming."

"I got held up by traffic."

"I just figured you weren't coming. In a way I wouldn't blame you."

"Hm," the volunteer asked, "why is that?"

"Well, here I am in this old geri chair and in this horrible nursing home. I can't walk, hardly move. I'm missing some teeth. Why would anyone want to visit me, anyone that didn't have to?"

"Because you're a fine person, a fine human being. And I enjoy seeing you."

Example: Mrs. A. B.

Mrs. A. B., an eighty-six-year-old widow and former secretary, was bothered by diabetes but was typically determined to a point of outward hardness. Yet she was a sensitive person who occasionally solicited support from others, and on this afternoon sought that from the volunteer. "But I don't suppose you have any idea how it is with an old person, a really old person. You know, one crippled up with several things, one who can hardly walk any more? You know, like me."

"You're right. I don't fully know your circumstance. Yet I do try, and I'm concerned about your well being, and I admire your determination and good spirit."

Mrs. A. B. eyed the volunteer carefully, making her judgment. "Okay, I can buy that, though I'm not quite sure of it. Yet you do come and see me and that stands for something good."

Active Listening

As a volunteer you must give the client your undivided attention, listen to what she says and how she says it, including her tone of voice, facial expression, gestures, posture, and movement of her body. Further, if she is silent, you may be aware, or have some idea about what she might be thinking and feeling. That is, you should be cognizant that she might be sending messages through her silence, facial expressions, and body gestures. Active listening requires discipline to remain silent and withhold comment and advice. It means not talking even though it makes you uncomfortable and edgy. Other skills of listening are: looking at the person while listening, giving complete attention to her, making occasional responses such as nodding, changing expressions to respond to hers, reflecting back a few leading words and asking a limited number of questions. Occasionally, you may check out what she has been saying by asking, "You are saying that . . . ?" "Do I understand you properly when I say . . . ?" Interrupting, if done at all, must be done very carefully, even when confusion reigns. Further, you must be tolerant and non-judgmental, which means no moralizing or condemning in any way.

Example: Mrs. W.

Mrs. W. was a seventy-six-year-old widow, a victim of a double stroke, whose right side was paralyzed. As a part of the paralysis, her right arm was turned upward and twisted in a peculiar manner. Given her condition, she was unable to move herself and spent most of her daily hours in a geri chair located in the day room of the nursing home, watching other patients, watching television, or looking out the windows. She was depressed about her situation and a number of things from the past, including the death of her father thirty years ago. After expressing her grief and complaining about her current condition, she "leveled off" and seemed moderately content.

Following this, she considered her previous career as a secretary and her contribution to the agency for which she worked. She alluded to her family occasionally; however, she never mentioned her deceased husband, who played a significant, though very troublesome, role in her later years, particularly immediately before she was admitted to the nursing home.

Her fragile nature suggested that inquiring about him should be delayed. Further, it was reasoned that Mrs. W. would broach the topic when she was ready. So the volunteer remained alert to the matter, listened and waited for several months as she dealt with a range of other subjects. She carefully avoided talking about her husband during that period.

Finally, as she was talking about one of her sisters who lived in Phoenix, she spontaneously said, "That's where I met Bill." It was the springboard for reviewing that relationship and its many problems.

Example: Mr. H. A.

Mr. H. A. was a seventy-nine-year-old-widower, crippled with arthritis that kept him from walking. So he spent considerable time in a wheelchair.

He was a former high school coach and reveled in talking about the exploits of his teams, and more than occasionally entertained his listeners with his exploits as an athlete.

This talk went on for a couple of months, and the volunteer listened with interest and asked questions occasionally to clarify a story or learn its relationship to other aspects of his life.

Mr. H. A. sensed the volunteer's interest and appreciated his patient, thoughtful listening. After the second month of telling his stories, Mr. H. A. slowed down, especially after he became aware of his repeating, and after contemplating, said, "You know, we never won the state championship. I've never been able to admit it, even face it. At first I was afraid to because of my job. You know, I was expected to win and win big. When I didn't, it didn't take long for criticism to come from the press, from the fans, and even from the school principal, who was supposed to be interested in academics. But he knew the public wanted a big-time high school team. So that's what he pushed, and he pushed me! I didn't like it but didn't feel I could fight it directly. So I gave it a deaf ear. But it all hurt. Let me tell you.

"Afterwards, you know, I retired from coaching and went into school administration. But even there I couldn't face my failure to win a state championship. I had to see myself as a big-time winner. That even got worse when I retired completely. I needed to look back to a rosier picture than I actually had painted. . . ." Mr. H. A.'s voice trailed, and he added, "Thank you for listening to me, including the sad part."

"Would you talk about it further? I sense you are still mulling it over."

Encouraging Expression

Part of the continuing contact with an elderly person is the client's expression—that is, her talking, recalling and reflecting on what she recalls; verbally exploring her immediate situation and past; and occasionally projecting the future. It may be demanding, given the limited health, intellectual acumen and interest of some clients. Yet clients should be encouraged to express themselves as fully as possible, as it provides them a sense of release, insight into themselves and their situation, and may increase their sense of personal worth.

Example: Mrs. H.

Mrs. H. was a seventy-seven-year-old widowed stroke victim who had difficulty in casting her thoughts into words. This was complicated by her self-consciousness about it. She would fret and say emphatically, "It makes me so mad!"

The volunteer encouraged her expression by: 1) listening patiently; 2) proceeding very slowly, in a relaxed manner; 3)waiting for her responses and being sure not to interrupt her or fill in for her when her sentences broke off; 4) maintaining a high level of interest in what she had to say; and 5) reassuring her occasionally about her delivery.

These procedures facilitated her communication, including the venting of anger and depression about the paralysis; however, first she speculated on when she was plagued by the paralysis.

"I know I didn't have it when I came here to the nursing home." (This was not true; rather, it was a memory distortion.)

"Do you recall when you were admitted?"

"About a year ago." (Which was correct.) "Maybe I got this way before I came."

"Hm . . . then it might have been before?"

She nodded her head. "I just don't know when it happened." Her expression became clouded with sadness. "I just know it makes me feel bad, real bad."

"Bad?"

"Sure," Mrs. H. replied caustically. "Here I am sitting or lying in this chair, can't move, or hardly move. Who wouldn't feel bad?" Tears came to her eyes. "I would just do anything to get out of here. I've had it here . . . with the place and the people."

"Here?"

"Sure, this chair and this place."

"It's good that you can say these things."

"Who wouldn't?" Mrs. H. said savagely. "My people aren't here. I don't see anybody, excepting those who are paid. The place stinks. The people are out of it, most of them. And I am worse off than most! And my future is black!"

The volunteer could see the spreading of a grey pallor around Mrs. H.'s mouth as she talked, and it became all encompassing when she stopped and laid her head back against the cushion in a deep frown. They sat in silence for several minutes. The volunteer nodded his head to convey his empathy; however, Mrs. H. remained grim and silent.

In an effort to tap her further thoughts, the volunteer simply said, "Yes."

This did not prompt Mrs. H.

After a further lapse, the volunteer encouraged further expression, "And you see your future as black?"

Sullen faced, Mrs. H. blinked as the volunteer repeated what she had reported, and then she spoke ever so quietly. "The grace of life will be blessed with the darkness of death."

The volunteer sat quietly and extended his hand to her.

Example: Mrs. T. L.

Mrs. T. L. was a seventy-nine-year-old former seamstress. Exacting and meticulous in character, Mrs. T. L. strove to report her ideas as clearly as possible. Yet her exactness limited her conversation, particularly her spontaneity. Moreover, she strove to be exceptionally positive, and she rationalized, "To be otherwise wouldn't do any good anyway." In this manner she avoided anything problematic or negative. Yet in her unguarded moments with nursing assistants, she complained vaguely about her deceased husband and their strained relationship, but did not explain further.

During that period the volunteer listened to her platitudes. He raised the possibility of other than positive experiences, as they are normal in everyday life. However, Mrs. T. L. rejected that suggestion.

Finally, in the third month of their visiting, Mrs. T. L.'s eyes twitched as she mentioned her husband, and the volunteer wondered whether some untoward feelings might surface; however, that did not happen. Rather, Mrs. T. L. fell silent, and an inquiry by the volunteer did not bring a response.

In the next, the twelfth, interview, her underlying concern broke through. "It's just gotten too much for me. Too much! I'm just going to have to tell you more about Henry and me. To begin, it wasn't all smooth by any measure. Not by any measure."

"I'm glad you're able to bring it out. Might you talk more about it?"

Talking-Sharing and Suggesting

Though a volunteer should mainly be a listener, there will be occasions where you will need to be more active and engage in sharing experiences and ideas, and on occasions suggesting or proposing ideas and/or actions to the elderly person.

Talking-Sharing

The strategy of listening, though the preferred way of working, has its outer limit because the elderly person will expect some reciprocity for her output. She will ask you about your activities, experiences, background and opinions. The exact manner of handling such requests will vary, depending on the client and the kind of questions that are asked. Generally, however, the client expects to hear substance from you beyond the minimal or token responses, which you may be inclined to offer in order to keep the focus on her. In such an instance the elderly person's disposition is to reject a minimal response or having her query reflected back to her. To make the most of the circumstance is to share a relevant experience openly and in good spirit, and limit it to that.

Example: Mrs. J.

Mrs. J. was a sixty-eight-year-old widowed stroke victim who had worked as a civilian secretary to the military in her youth. Afflicted with a paralysis, accompanying speech difficulties and characteristic shyness made it difficult for her to talk. However, after getting acquainted she spoke about an assignment to Vienna, Austria. She enjoyed the station but was upset by the army's rigid bureaucracy and felt subordinated.

She accepted the volunteer's empathy and talked, though very slowly and brokenly, of her frustration and intimidation. She gritted her teeth and looked directly at the volunteer. "You must have been up against that kind of thing. Sometimes."

Initially the volunteer encouraged her to talk more about her frustration. This response did not meet with success. He then attempted to learn about her motivation for the query, and she responded, "You want me to do all the talking but sometimes you have to say something too. Say something."

The volunteer attempted, "I know exactly what you are talking about. I was in the military for three years. Rules came down the line from above.

That's where the higher ranks and authority were, and there was very little one could do— maybe nothing—to change it. I know what you mean." Mrs. J. smiled.
"At least you were a civilian and could leave if you decided it was too much. I didn't have that choice."
Mrs. J. laughed.

Example: Mr. F.

Mr. F. was a ninety-three-year-old nursing home resident who was motivated to visit; however, he was seriously limited by a stroke, an early dementia, and bouts with depression.

On one occasion, he recalled reroofing a building during a very hot summer day. He repeated this experience several times, obviously enjoying it, grimacing, and then empathically mentioned the camaraderie among the roofers and himself. Despite his success in articulating the experience, Mr. F. stopped, threw his hands upward in great dismay, and shook his head, indicating the inability to carry the thought any further, and his speech faltered as he tried.

The volunteer's attempts to help him continue, first by repeating his verbalization in the hope that he would pick it up, failed. He then asked Mr. F. some direct questions, but to no avail. After waiting for a prolonged period, Mr. F. haltingly asked, "Did you ever, did you ever, did you ever . . . do anything like it, like it?"

"No," the volunteer replied, "not quite like it, but I spent some extremely hot days in the wheat fields of Kansas, and I know exactly what you were talking about."

Mr. F. smiled and nodded his head with satisfaction.

Suggesting

Your suggestions may help the elderly person if she is forgetful and has difficulty keeping track of things, including her ideas. Such suggestions are reminders. Suggestions may be also used to provide alternatives for the elderly person to consider in making decisions. They may broaden her range of choices on such elementary procedures as selecting activities to attend, deciding which projects to undertake, and writing to friends and relatives. Suggestions also may help the client understand herself and her experience, especially the possible meanings of what she says, or holds back. Such suggestions, however, must be made sparingly and gently, and be based on a firm, positive relationship. To do otherwise is likely to result in having the suggestions rejected and is likely to disturb the client.

Suggesting, under any circumstances, does not mean ordering or directing the client's every move, and certainly does not mean being authoritarian or officious. Moreover, as has been indicated, it should be done only occasionally and discreetly to protect the client's initiative and self-determination.

Example: Mr. T.

Mr. T. was a seventy-four-year-old arthritic widower whose mental functioning was impaired by a dementia. However, his basic intelligence was very good. He tended to be positive, yet impulsive and emotionally labile. Moreover, he was reluctant to participate in any of the nursing home's activities or converse with others. In spite of his stand-off disposition, he was reluctantly friendly, and generally was in a good mood.

The volunteer had seen him for several weeks, and all the while he maintained a stand-off style, complaining about the aloofness of others and the lack of anything to do. On a particular day soon thereafter he continued to complain about his lack of friends. The volunteer intervened. "I suggest that you select one person, maybe two, with whom you would like to spend a bit of time. Talk with them, joke a bit, go to an activity together, hang out together, even if it's just watching TV, and the first thing you know you may have a friend. Continue it and you may have two or three."

"Well, I don't really know about that," Mr. T. responded unenthusiastically.

"Why not?"

"I just don't know."

"You're a likable person. They'll respond."

Mr. T. shrugged.

"Again, I suggest it."

"I really don't know," Mr. T. continued. However, his resistance had weakened, and he added, "Well . . ."

"Mr. T., we can talk about your reluctance as times goes on, try to understand it, and so on. But right now you really need to move off of dead center, and I'll help you."

Mr. T. was struck by the volunteer's language. "Do you really mean that?"

"Sure."

"Well, maybe I should try to do something, make some kind of move. I hadn't mentioned it, but I did have a conversation with Mr. E. down in the corner room the other day. Maybe I'll follow up."

"Why not?"

Example: Mrs. B.

Mrs. B. was a sixty-year-old widow whose arthritis had crippled her knees and put her in a wheelchair. Though passive, she participated in the nursing home program. Yet because of her shyness and passiveness, she failed to make friends and therefore was lonely in an institution of people. She had talked about this problem for a time, but mainly complained, without taking any initiative to change the circumstance.

She was a fragile person, so the volunteer gently suggested, "Have you ever considered zeroing in on this matter, either to talk about it in some depth or to act on it immediately, that is, do something other than talk?"

"Oh yes, I've tried to make friends. I really have, but . . ."

"But . . . ?"

"It just isn't easy. People don't just do how you want them to."

"How is that?"

"A couple of weeks ago I asked a couple of people to stop by after the movie. And they said, 'Sorry, we can't do it tonight. Maybe some other night.' Well, since I put myself out, I thought they would invite me back, but they didn't."

"And you gave up?"

Mrs. B. nodded. "What's the use?"

"Might you try again?"

"Well, not those two. Maybe somebody else."

"Do you have any specific plans?"

Mrs. B. shook her head.

After a pause the volunteer followed, "Seems like it's worth a try. You'd be an attractive friend. I feel they would respond."

Mrs. B. did not answer but looked to the floor.

"Were your feelings hurt?"

Mrs. B. nodded. "I just thought they could have been nicer."

"I doubt they meant to hurt you in any way. I suggest you give it another try, really. If not with those two people, then with somebody else."

"Well, if you think I can do it, I'll try."

Persisting

It is all too easy, but incorrect, to believe that all elderly persons, including those who are isolated and lonely, want to talk about the pleasantries and problems of the day, delve into their past, and project the future. This assumption overlooks the precariousness of the elder's adjustment, the anxiety that is associated with talking about problems and uncertainties, and the person's cognitive limitations.

They may have detached themselves from the past, at least as much as they can, and you may encounter, "Oh, I don't know. Really I don't. That was so long, long ago. I can't remember." And they may reject the present because it offers so few satisfactions and too many affronts. Likewise, the future may be avoided because it is too ominous.

Additionally, if weighted down by the preoccupation with death and dying and an unwillingness to share it, clients may restrict their participation in talking and, in some instances, remain mute during most of your time with them.

Such a challenge requires your persistence, optimism and affirmation of the aged person. Also, a reexamination of the elderly person may be in order and the techniques and goals that have been pursued in her behalf.

Another scenario may challenge you. It pertains to an elderly person's progressive dementia, progressing to the point where her language is impaired to unintelligible mumbling, or near mumbling, from a previous reasonable articulation. At that point, you may have to change your manner of communicating with her by sensing very carefully the emotions she conveys in her mumbling, and mirroring back these emotions through facial expressions and gestures, as well as trying to pick up any verbal messages that she may give.

Example: Mrs. A.

Mrs. A. was a seventy-two-year-old stroke victim who also had the early signs of a dementia. All of this was superimposed on a basic hysterical personality.

Her forgetfulness and slight confusion, combined with her play-acting, emotional liability and anxiety, produced shifting thoughts and moods during the first three visits. Her response to the direction of talking about whatever was important to her included: "What could I possibly talk about? I can't even think about anything important."

Given that she did not speak at the beginning of the fourth visit, and her general forgetfulness, the volunteer was prompted to gently reaffirm his earlier suggestion, "Tell me about yourself, what's been important to you. Anything you like, for example, the activities in your daily life. Or some of your experiences of your childhood, growing up. Whatever you choose." Surprisingly, Mrs. A. began to relay, though haltingly, aspects of her career as a biochemist, her relationship to her deceased husband, and visits with friends. Before the time concluded, the volunteer complimented her, "You did an excellent job of talking about yourself and what's important to you. Why don't we continue next week."

Example: Mrs. Mc.

Mrs. Mc. was an eighty-two-year-old widowed stroke victim who walked haltingly with the assistance of a cane. She lived in an apartment with the help of a nursing assistant eight hours a day. She spent her evenings and nights alone. She read the daily paper in detail and worked the crossword puzzles with determination.

Independent, self-contained and rigid, she said very little to the volunteer, though she was generally polite. But there wasn't anything spontaneous about her. After fifteen or twenty minutes she usually suggested that it was time for the volunteer to leave, which the volunteer honored. This pattern continued for several months until one day Mrs. Mc. smiled in a reserved manner and matter-of-factly began, "I thought you'd go away by now, but you haven't. So I would like you to know how it was that I became a teacher."

Teaching

Teaching takes place in helping work, but it is not classroom teaching. It is more subtle, informal, surely less direct, and only occasional.

You have two jobs as a teacher. The first one is to advise the elderly person about the elementary procedures of the relationship. This undertaking may be a bit more complex than it appears because it asks the elderly person to commit herself to a relationship by giving time and thought, and being candid. This means you must extend yourself, in addition to being someone to reach out to.

It is your task to tell the elderly person this to begin with, and then gently and clearly carry through. The elderly person, given her life-long habits, may proceed down a different pathway, and have to be reminded that she is expected to talk about whatever is important to her. This technique is partly done by demonstration and practice along with the instruction. After telling her about the procedures for the interviews, you may follow with questions such as, "So, what have you been thinking about during the past week?" Assuming the elderly person discloses some of her thoughts, you may try for a more detailed picture by asking such questions as, "And what all was involved?" "Does any of that tie to what you have been thinking recently?"

Oftentimes current experiences and concerns relate to past ones. For example, the feelings of sadness over a recent family member's death is related to the unresolved despondency over an earlier family member's death. As a part of the teaching process, you should help the client understand that past and current experiences often relate to each other.

Example: Mrs. D. O.

Mrs. D. O. was a mentally alert, melodramatic seventy-four-year-old widow who was confined to a wheelchair because of a stroke. She also had a history of alcoholism. Hysterical-like, she tended to be impulsive, exclaiming on matters having any emotion associated with them, and playing out thoughts in pantomime manner, which she could not complete because of a stroke-caused speech difficulty. At the nursing home she refused to attend physical therapy and all leisure activities excepting happy hour. Her condition was compounded by an early dementia.

During the eighth visit she went through her typical routine: "It's so terrible here. There's nothing to do here. The new patients get all the attention. Nobody cares. I'd like to get out of here." She concluded by raising her eyebrows, throwing her head back, rolling her eyes and asking "What would you do?"

Many efforts had been made to enroll her in the home's activities: having nursing assistants take her; urging her to accept the responsibility to take herself; bringing certain activities — for example, crafts — to her room. However, they all failed because she rejected them.

As she continued to complain in subsequent sessions, the volunteer asked, "What are you going to do?"

But it was to no avail. She rolled her eyes and threw her hands up in the air.

This was followed by attempts to teach Mrs. D. O. to be more reflective. The volunteer encouraged, "Take your time. Think it over. Give yourself a chance to consider various ways to get to and do some of the activities. Plan every move. Think them out in your mind. Think over what you are going to say, and how you're going to say it. Practice all of this in your room. That's the way to go after it."

She threw her hands into the air again and the volunteer responded, "Relax and give yourself a chance, think over exactly what you want to do and what you want to say. When you get that organized, don't hold back. Just say it."

She nodded her head, raised her eyebrows, and haltingly said something distant from the volunteer's suggestion. "Oh my God! The thought is a picture of me and my husband on a vacation at the lake . . . and now I'm in here!"

The volunteer was moved by her response. "That was a great memory. Any details on it?"

"That's it."

"Give it more of a try. Think about it."

"Well, it was great. We used to go there every summer if we could manage it."

"You must have enjoyed it."

"Oh, yes. We would stay a week or two. Just take it easy. Swim and do things like that."

Mrs. D. O. stopped and the volunteer encouraged, "You can pull important memories together. You just did."

Mrs. D. O. smiled, "Well, okay," and then threw her hands into the air, shrugged her shoulders to discount the achievement.

However, the volunteer countered, "You did it. Clearly you did it. Now, what activity will you go to this week? Let's plan the detailed steps for that."

Example: Mrs. P.

Mrs. P. was a seventy-year-old widow who had diabetes and was incontinent. Though she was bright and had an engaging sense of humor, her thoughts and conversation often meandered. Consequently, the visits with her were friendly but unfocused and sometimes nearly without substance and overall significance.

To bring more connections into the conversation the volunteer encouraged, "Mrs. P., might you consider tracking your ideas just a bit more?" This suggestion came in the course of good rapport, and Mrs. P.

raised her eyebrows with a note of exaggerated exasperation and laughed. "I can't do it, really. Can you teach me?"

"I can teach you to have confidence in your ability to attend and concentrate. So I say to you right now, I know you can do it. I've heard you do it in the past, and quite well." Gently the volunteer furthered, "Give it a try."

"Okay, okay."

With that, Mrs. P. made an effort. "Yes, after my husband died I found myself free of a lot of hassle, more financially secure, but lonesome. Lonesome."

The volunteer encouraged Mrs. P. to explore the lonesomeness, which she then did with help from the volunteer as he suggested and helped her articulate her situation.

Normalizing

In the course of your volunteering, you may conclude that the client is a basically strong, intact person who has encountered difficult times in the past, but who was able to handle them successfully. Given that as the case, you may strive to normalize the difficulties the client may present; that is, to interpret them as being regrettable but normal in the course of life, and her reactions to them as being normal, whether it be grief over a loss or anxiety over the threat of a medical procedure. In so doing, you will use common cultural or community interpretations to explain the strains she may be experiencing.

Example: Mrs. X.

Mrs. X. was a soft-spoken, gentle widow of seventy-seven who typically avoided or denied any disturbing matter. Despite having a serious heart problem and being frail, she could walk without assistance in the nursing home. Excepting for talking with several women from her hometown, she kept to herself, even when in the day room. The husband of one of these women died abruptly, and that greatly upset Mrs. X.

The dynamics of her disturbance were not clear. Was her upset due to sympathy for her friend? Did it ignite the unresolved grief about her own husband? Was it some combination of these? The volunteer did not want to exacerbate the woman's grief about her husband. So he provided empathy and psychological support and interpreted her sadness as sympathy for her friend. Mrs. X. accepted the volunteer's efforts and was back to her usual self in about two months.

Example: Mr. E. M.

Mr. E. M. was a seventy-six-year-old arthritic patient. Though confined to a wheelchair, he moved about the nursing home with ease, visited other patients and participated in activities. However, his wife, who was also in the nursing home, become deathly ill with cancer, and died. Mr. E. M. was devastated and became tearful at any mention of the topic. The volunteer listened, empathized and pointed out that his grieving was natural. He and his wife had been part of each other's life for over fifty years. He loved her dearly, and he would surely miss her. But time would clearly ease the grief. Repetition of this theme and support over a period of several months helped move Mr. E. M. back to his previous self.

Reviewing, Clarifying, Focusing

You, in your role of volunteer, may ask the client to repeat a matter of importance in order to sharpen, complete, or focus an idea that may be lost in a welter of thoughts or, more simply, to hear what has been said, but said in an inaudible voice. This helps to firm up the conversation and helps you understand the concern of the elderly person. It also may enable the elderly person to become aware of a previously overlooked or denied matter. This technique may also help the elderly person trace the relationship of one item to another item, and suggest the next steps to be taken.

Reviewing and Clarifying

Example: Mrs. N.

Mrs. N. was a seventy-year-old stroke victim, a widow and former secretary. After talking about her father briefly, she shifted to recounting day-to-day activities at the nursing home, and then cautiously shifted back to her father and spoke of his death and aspects of his parenting. "It was bad, real bad to see him go. He carried the family. But he was strict, especially when it came to going out with boys. That's where he wouldn't let me go out with anybody, none of the boys my age, and for sure not with a teacher."
"A teacher?"

"I was in a special math class, one in which the better students were, and the teacher was young, real young, nice and all, and he asked if he could take me to a movie in Baltimore. That was about twenty miles from home. I didn't answer yes or no but went home and asked my mother, who passed it on to my dad. Well, he said, 'In no way, no.' I felt bad but didn't say anything back."

"You felt that you couldn't say anything back?"

"That is right. He was the boss in the family. And though I didn't like what he said, I couldn't do anything about it."

"Were there any further developments on that?"

"No, I figured the teacher made his try and when he didn't succeed, he left me out as a possible girlfriend."

"Might you have talked further with your father? I sense he was the authority in your family."

"That's right, but I didn't. He was gruff and short, and always figured he was right. We didn't give him any trouble. It was sad how he died. I don't know what he had. We had such poor medical help. He just wasted away one winter. It wasn't too long and we knew he was going, and on March fifteenth he died."

"Yes."

"Well, it was hard. We all loved him. Besides, we were poor. That's when we kids all went out and got whatever work we could."

Example: Mrs. U.

Mrs. U. was a stroke victim, in her seventies, and a reclusive person. Yet on the second contact she became tearful, but was hesitant to say what was bothering her until the volunteer said, "I know you feel badly, I can feel it myself." She looked at him, and he nodded with understanding.

Then, amid gasps of crying she said, "I've never gotten over the passing of my mother, my older sister and my younger brother. It's been some time ago but I miss them so."

As Mrs. U. continued to cry, the volunteer gave her a tissue and commented, "I'm sure it is hard for you, and good of you to say so, to get it out."

Mrs. U. then began to talk about their deaths. It was never clear as to who she was grieving.

The volunteer tried, "Might you consider just one person at a time? It seems you had several people together."

Mrs. U. nodded and began to cry. "My mother."

Focusing

Example: Mrs. E. B.

Mrs. E. B., an alert, seventy-seven-year-old widow slowed down seriously by arthritis, had talked considerably about her only daughter, with whom she had a poor relationship. Yet Mrs. E. B. never focused on the essence of their relationship. Instead, she complained about her daughter: headstrong courtship and poor marriage; extravagance, especially on clothes; inconsistent parenting of her young daughter; failure to visit; and lack of maturity, poor judgment and personal insensitivity. Yet, after making these charges she played them down by laughing, throwing up her hands, and commenting, "I guess she'll learn in time."

After listening to another of these episodes, the volunteer said, "In talking about your daughter`s behavior for the past several weeks, I sense you're avoiding something. You seem to be skirting around something."

"Oh sure, something that had happened a long time ago."

"Can you focus on it?"

"Well, if you want the truth, I never wanted her in the first place. She was forced on me, first by my boyfriend who became my husband, and then my parents who wouldn't let me get an abortion! That's the bald truth, and let me tell you more! I never would have married Lenny if I hadn't been pregnant by him. And my parents were putting on the pressure. Now you know the rock bottom truth!"

Mrs. E. B.'s revelation was aggressively stated, and the volunteer matter-of-factly suggested, "You have been carrying that a long, long time."

"Too long. Too long. It should have been said years ago, but I didn't have the guts to say so. Figured the roof would come down! Even now I'm afraid the roof might come down."

"On whom?"

"On me, because my daughter might find out. Think how badly she will feel to know all this."

"I surely won't tell, and I sense you won't either."

"No way! No way!"

"And your parents and your husband have passed away."

"I know. I know. But . . . ?"

Mrs. E. B. was not only rough around the edges, but something very rough was lodged deeply at the center. She was a complicated, selfish, harsh, yet a lonely woman.

"You're still concerned about your daughter finding out?"

"Sure, that's it."

"I don't understand you. Let me run the main points by you again, then you tell me how your daughter will learn the facts."

The irrationality of Mrs E. B.'s reasoning was played out as the interview continued. Specifically, she discovered that her intense anger towards the daughter was driving her to inform the daughter (against her better judgment) of this regrettable piece of history. She was driven by the madness, in spite of herself.

As the interview continued, and it continued for some considerable length, the anger was partially discharged and the volunteer felt that Mrs. E. B. would contain herself.

Example: Mr. T. A.

"Can you pull it together?" the volunteer encouraged Mr. T. A., an eighty-four-year-old resident of a group home who had difficulty remembering.

Not discouraged, Mr. T. A. continued, "Let me try. Now I know my being in Canada had something to do with my wife's death. . . . Now, if you'll just give me a minute. . . ."

"I'm with you. Can you bring it up and connect it to your move?"

"Well, let me see. I'll get it."

After a pause Mr. T. A. asked, "What was your question? Did it have to do with my move to Canada?"

"That's right. You're right on it."

"I rightfully don't know, but if I had to guess, it had to do with finding a place to live after my wife died. And I did have a daughter up there."

Summarizing

Somewhat like *Reviewing*, *Clarifying*, *Focusing*, concise summarizing by you may be used in several ways: to give the client the theme of her verbalizations and thereby give her the opportunity to draw the relationships among them, or give her a place from which to continue. Such may be done at any time, including at the beginning or conclusion of a session.

Also, summarizing is a technique to assist in terminating a helping relationship should the client not need any further assistance, or if you are unable to continue, or if the client decides to discontinue. Summing up is a way of pulling the main features of the experience together, and should allow the client full opportunity to express her disappointment and anger, if such are involved. Transfer to a successor should be arranged before you depart, if transferring is the plan.

Example: Mrs. R.

After seven months, Mrs. R. introduced her deceased husband into the conversation. In the course of the next several visits she entertained several possibilities about his being alive or dead, and his whereabouts if alive. She seriously considered each of the possibilities as she iterated them. Her health problems were many: stroke with serious paralysis, early dementia, and paranoid aspects to her thinking.

In reality he was dead and his remains were with a Washington, D.C. mortuary. The following characterized her preoccupation: "I know he's not dead. He's too ornery to be dead. Might even be in jail. He didn't always do what was right." On a less humorous note she added, "I think he's on a secret mission for the CIA, or the FBI, maybe the military, and can't write to me. Yet, he may be dead. You know those undercover missions are dangerous, and the government won't even tell you what's happened. I've been told he's buried in Arizona, and I asked for his body to be shipped here but they won't do it. I just know he's not dead because he visited me daily just a couple of months ago."

"Mrs. R., you have spoken about several possibilities. Where do you stand on the matter?"

"I just don't believe he's dead."

"The record says he's dead. I know that's harsh, but that's what it says. And his remains are in a mortuary in Washington."

"I know that is what they say, but I don't believe it. And I don't want you to check into it any more. It could be dangerous."

"How is that?"

"Because he might have been on some CIA mission and was killed. They aren't going to want anybody looking into it. And if you get too nosy they'll get you too!"

"So after you look over the several possibilities and the facts, where do you come out on this?"

"He's alive."

"Sure?"

"That's right."

Mrs. R. held onto her delusion for months in the future.

Example: Mr. R. P.

Mr. R. P. was a highly intelligent, seventy-seven-year-old arthritic person who was known as a "talker" among his friends at the nursing home. The volunteer had difficulty following his talk as he shifted from event to event, covering very different times of his life. To bring focus to their visiting the volunteer asked, "How can we get the several items of your interest together? That is, how might they relate to each other?"

"Oh, sure. Sure, I can do that. No problem. Like I was saying. . . ."

"Let me summarize. You have spoken about a variety of things: about your grade and high school subjects related to engineering, about your college course in electrical engineering, and working at GE. Along the way you mentioned an uncle or two, your father and a special high school girlfriend."

Mr. R. P. nodded.

"If that's a fair summary, might you say a bit more of the uncles and your father in these events?"

Spiritual Matters

Many elderly emphasize the spiritual part of their lives, or are concerned about it. Such may be the continuation of an earlier way of life. Or it may be prompted by a recent concern about their mortality. Under any circumstance, they seek a deeper significance of their lives and their place in the world and in the hereafter. Also, physical limitations, frailty, or the threat of a debilitating illness or a terminal disease may stimulate spiritual interests.

Meditation and prayer may guide the elderly person's search for spiritual strength, particularly as they stem from religious beliefs and convictions. Early faith or more recently developed convictions may encourage the spiritual quest of the person.

You must be sensitive to the elderly person's spiritual interests. Further, you must be receptive to whatever the person has to say or preoccupies her, and be tolerant and non-judgmental. The overall aim is affirm the person's sense of well being. If the interests and/or concerns are beyond your competence, consultation of the clergy should be sought. It may be for the client, or you, or both.

A Proactive Stance: Facilitating the Life Review Process

Narrowly defined, a life review is a spontaneous, self-directed recall of pertinent life experiences, particularly earlier ones, by elderly people in their intuitive interest of integrating those experiences with more recent ones. They seek a refined, if not a totally clear, perspective on their life. Though mainly a cognitive experience, a life review also involves a range of emotions as, for example, joy as happy events are recalled and dismay as traumas are drawn upon.

More broadly, a life review may be deliberately elicited, that is, called forth by a volunteer. Resistances such as avoidance and denial by a client are common. They stand in front of traumas and conflicts. You must help the client work through the resistances in order to get at the more basic problems that underlie them.

Such a broader review may be initiated soon after you develop a relationship with the client, particularly if you believe the direction and structure of a life review will provide her guidelines for responding and therein offer some security. Or it may be attempted later if the client is unable to respond to a more open-ended interviewing.

With the exception of spontaneous, self-directed life reviews, most review procedures provide the client with a format to follow, for example, beginning with the client's earliest memories, followed by her preschool and elementary school activities, then her secondary school, college and early work experiences. Also, the format will ask about her dating, courtship, marriage and family life (if she married and had a family), about her career, and later life experience.

Many of the person's recollections will be saturated by interpersonal relationships—with family, friends, lovers, enemies—and reflect a range of emotions, ranging from joy to sorrow. Though you may strive to work forward systematically from the client's early childhood to her senior years, such may not work out that neatly. The elderly person responds in her own unique way, often mixing various periods in her life, or emphasizing one aspect and neglecting others. Yet you must allow the person to develop her own pattern. Besides affording the client the freedom to tell her story in her own way, her choice and arrangement of substance will indicate what is important to her and may offer clues as to what she avoids.

The life story approach, when elicited by you, is likely to be more problem-oriented than one generated by an elderly person spontaneously. You must be particularly sensitive to problems if you seek to help the client talk them through with the ultimate aim of enhancing her happiness.

Example: Mrs. J. B. (Only brief parts of her life review are given because of space limitations.)

The following example of a life review was initiated in the fourth meeting with the client, Mrs. J. B., because she had difficulty focusing her thoughts. She responded to the procedure; however, the editing of her reflections gives them greater continuity, clarity and organization than they had in fact. Some of her speech difficulties and perseveration, though reported, are under-reported to avoid repetition. Its editing reduced the length of the review substantially. However, the substance is consistent with her recollections.

Several points in her history stand out, that is, had significant emotions attached to them: regrets about her selection of college and spouse, the death of her brother, husband, and Aunt Julia, her bout with alcoholism, her dissatisfaction with life in the nursing home, earlier difficulties at school, and family stress related to her father's business reverses.

A seventy-nine-year-old widow and former high school teacher, Mrs. J. B. was restricted to a wheelchair because of permanent injuries incurred in an auto accident. She was intelligent, and though she had an occasional "down," her morale was generally good, and she thrived on a good sense of humor. Her condition, however, was complicated by the signs of a dementia and an aphasia-like speech problem. Mrs. J. B. attempted to compensate for her speech problem by playing out her ideas through dramatic facial expressions, body movements and arm and hand gestures.

Excerpts from Early Childhood

"So . . . so . . . you want me to talk about my earliest memories, . . . memories from way back?"

"That's right."

"Don't, don't you have an easier assignment? . . . I don't know if I can do that, really. . . . No."

"Why not give it a try, a good one."

"Well . . . let's see. This goes way back. . . . I must have been three or four. I guess four. There was a lot of excitement in the house because it was my . . . my birthday!"

"What was happening?"

"I guess it was a party. Yes, . . . a party for me, for me. And I was all dressed up, and I think it was a Sunday and a lot of the relatives were over, and . . . everybody was making a fuss over me."

"Hm."

"I don't remember anything else, excepting we had ice cream. That was right down to what I liked. . . . That's about it."

"Fine, fine. Might you reach back just a bit further?"

"I don't know. . . . Well, I can say one other thing, . . . and that's about it. It was some time before my party. Yes maybe six or seven months, . . . maybe a year earlier. That's when my brother was born. You know, he was born right in the house, in my parents' bed. None of that hospital stuff . . . that we have now. He was born right there in the house, and he got along fine. At least that's what I've heard. . . . I was born right in the same place. . . . 'Course I don't remember that!"

"Your brother's birth was important."

Mrs. J. B. talked about the long and positive relationship with her brother and cried when she mentioned his death, which had occurred five or six years before the life review.

Excerpt from Preschool Years

"Not much that I remember right off. No . . . I was home with my mother, and little brother, played in the neighborhood. I had a good friend, Lora, just a couple houses up the street. Yes, she was a year older than me and had brothers and sisters in school. So, so she told me all about the first grade. I was ready to go when I was only five. We didn't have a kindergarten. I was keyed up to go. Excited and all. My mother taught me some things at home. Yes, she taught me at home. I guess I was ready, and she wanted to be sure I would do well. I had my numbers in mind and could count to a hundred and could do a little reading, not much, but some. All before I started school."

"And was your father working?"

"Yes, yes. He really worked hard. He was in the insurance business. So he was always seeing people, including some nights when he went to people's houses when both the man and wife were home, to sell them insurance."

"And what was your mother about?"

"What do you mean, what, what was she about?" Mrs. J. B. threw her hands up in the air and consternation appeared on her face.

"What kinds of things did she do?"

"She did a lot of things. Mother got us all to church on Sunday, and afterwards we would have a big Sunday dinner. She worked hard, but not much was happening then. Oh yes, there is one thing that comes back to me. My Aunt Julia died when I was five, or about then. She was my mother's older sister, and they were real close."

Mrs. J. b. grieved the death of her aunt and reminisced about the good times she had as a child at her home.

Excerpts from Early School Years

"Now you want me to talk about my first years in school. That will be easier, easier, than trying to remember some of that earlier stuff. Gee, let's see. Right off, I'll start with my first day at school. Everybody had talked about it, built it up—my mother, my dad, even my little brother, and my friend Lora. So I was all charged up to go. And I went . . . and I went, all by myself. The school was only a couple of blocks from where we lived. I was excited or maybe scared. I don't know which, maybe both. I walked right into the school building, and after some mistakes, got to the right room. Oh, the teacher was so nice! She put her arm around me, gave me a seat and all. And I was underway. Everything went well that day. . . . It just stands out in my mind. I rushed home after school and couldn't say enough to my mother, and my dad when he came home, he got the same business from me. Then there was my little brother taking it all in."

"Were all your first grade days as good as the first one?"

"No, I can't say they were, but I liked school, got along okay and had friends. No . . . I can't say they were. Especially when I got to the sixth grade, and there I had a teacher who treated everybody badly, the whole class. So I was included. I didn't like her. To be honest, I hated her!"

Mrs. J. B. talked at some length about her mixed grade school experience, some good teachers and some poor; however, on balance mostly good, and her experience was enjoyable.

Excerpts from High School and College

"High school wasn't exactly a breeze, but it wasn't very difficult either. I took the harder courses—math, sciences and languages. I wanted to go to college, and so I was getting ready for it. Now, now there were some teachers who were really great, then there were a few so-so ones. I really had one stinker, Mr. A., the physics teacher. He not only wanted you to believe that physics was the greatest subject in the world, but that he also was the world's greatest teacher. Well, he wasn't; what he was was right-down petty. You know, he counted off a fraction of a point on your answer even if you had the main idea. And he would put you down in front of the whole class, make you feel badly, and embarrass you. If he had any chance, he would be sure to do it. Every time! He was always looking for a kid who was most easily hurt. He picked on me, just once in a while, less than some of the others for sure. I survived because I stayed clear of him. He didn't have any respect from the kids, and I sure didn't show him any. Let's get onto something else. I had enough of him then and now." She shook her head, grimaced and asked, "What else have you got?"

Mrs J. B. described her several high school activities, then spent time on the failure of her father's business and its negative effects on the family, which included her being limited to a local college, a major disappointment.

Dating, which included several intense but short relationships, turned her to a blander relationship with a long-time friend whose parents were friends of her parents. Mrs. J. B. described him as "serious, a good student with the promise of a fine future. I liked him, but I never loved him. I was comfortable with him and my parents liked him. That's how that went. I have often thought my marriage was like my choice of a college. It wasn't great but it worked out fine."

Excerpts from Early and Mid-Adulthood

"We really had a big wedding! My parents wanted to give me a great send-off, and Bill's parents had the same feeling. They threw same money into it. I don't remember how much, but it was more than they could afford. It was a great show, and I showed my appreciation, did all the right things, said the right things, but down deep I wasn't real happy because I really didn't want to marry Bill. Not down deep I didn't, no.

"Well, anyway, Bill got into insurance and I taught. We made out real well financially. We got along with our families and visited a lot. We belonged to the country club and had friendly neighbors. They belonged too. We partied a lot. Too much."

Mrs. J. B. discussed her bouts with alcohol, her disappointment in not being able to have a family and regret about her marriage. She wept considerably in relating this period of her life.

Excerpts from Later Life

"I got here (nursing home) because my luck ran out. Like I said, Bill died, I drank too much, had an automobile accident, got crippled up and my mind was playing tricks on me. It was giving out, seemed like. I just can't remember like I used to, but it still works good enough for me to get along. I haven't lost my marbles! No. No . . . but I don't like it here. There is nothing to do. Nobody cares. I want something to do. What I really want to do is to go back to Baltimore. I want to get a job in the funeral home that buried my parents and Bill. I could arrange the flowers there. I could direct and help people as they come for funerals or to view the body." Mrs. J. B. shifted in her chair and stared at the ceiling. Apart from the immediate situation, her thoughts seemed to rise upwards with her stare. Preoccupied, she did not speak.

Mrs. J. B.'s dissatisfaction with the nursing home was her preoccupation for some time, and while she never reconciled herself to living there, she recognized the unrealism of working in the community. Also, she gained an appreciation that her dissatisfaction with the nursing home was associated with her life dissatisfactions.

Suggesting a Referral

A client may need a referral for recreational or social services, or a physical or a mental examination or laboratory tests based in part on your observations.

The complaints of the elderly person or other indications for further assistance should be brought to the attention of the charge nurse or responsible person, if the client is in a nursing home or some other setting. Your observations may corroborate the information they already have, or in some instances it may be new to them. In any case, clear reporting of the client's needs is essential.

In the realm of mental health, several symptoms require the attention of specialized help. You may or may not be prepared to deal with them. Minimally, you must bring the symptomatic behavior to the attention of the persons indicated above. If they already know the problem, you need to corroborate the information and learn what they have in mind for the client, help them with the client's daily care, and perhaps make a referral to a mental health specialist. To illustrate, a referral should be made if you are not prepared to deal with the following.

- If the client is unable to identify herself or where she is; cannot give the date or community in which she lives or recall events of the past 24 hours.
- If the client is seriously depressed, agitated, and restless, is apathetic, immobile, unable to arouse herself, mutilates herself, won't/can't care for herself, and doesn't eat, drink, bathe, or change clothes, and repeats ritualistic acts.
- If the client hallucinates — hears voices, sees visions: or has unverified bodily sensations; says her body feels unreal; fears losing her mind; shows extreme pressure of speech, and talks endlessly.
- If the client talks of killing herself.

Example: Mr. I. C.

A steady, even-tempered, seventy-eight-year-old intellectual describes Mr. I. C. He had very little in common with the other residents in a group home. He was lonesome but passive with other residents and staff and did not reach out.

Observing this, the volunteer asked him to consider entering a day activity program at a nearby nursing home one or more days a week, whatever he might choose. However, after listening to the proposal, Mr. I. C. quietly said, "No. I don't think so." Convinced of the activity's value, the volunteer urged it. However, Mr. I. C. rejected it. "No, I don't think I will find anyone there with common interests."

Not giving up, the volunteer suggested, "Consider it. You won't really know its quality until you try it. I'll go with you the first time or two if you like. I'm sure you'll find some congenial persons there."

Mr. I. C. shook his head. The volunteer persisted, "Keep it in mind. You may want to consider it in the future."

Special Considerations

Relatives and Friends

The area of the family is a complex one. Its earlier, fuller make-up of parents and growing children may be reduced to consisting of solely a widow or widower. Surviving children and perhaps relatives may remain interested in the elderly person. However, such is not always the case.

The complexity of the family goes beyond who makes up a family and includes feelings—anger, jealousy, joy, love and hate—that are attached to the various relationships and may have long histories, including aggravations. One or several of these feelings may influence or dominate the manner in which a spouse, adult children and others respond to the elderly person.

The elderly person's condition—physical, psychological, economic—may be burdensome to others. Yet not all relations between the elderly and their significant others are problematic. Whatever positives remain of the elderly person's network of family and friends need to be sustained, particularly if they can help support the elderly person psychologically or materially.

Guardians, lawyers, social workers and the court may come into play as family and friends are not able to sustain an elderly person.

Example: Mrs. L. E.

Alzheimer's plagued Mrs. L. E., a seventy-four-year-old widow. Yet she retained some memory functioning, self-identity and awareness, though these attributes were diminishing.

Mrs. A. C., Mrs. L. E.'s sister, was ten years her junior, and had been raised in a different family than Mrs. L. E. She maintained an ambivalent attitude toward Mrs. L. E., perhaps generated by their different backgrounds. She rotated between lack of interest and over-concern. On one occasion, she insisted the nursing home place Mrs. L. E. into a rocker, comforted by pillows and strapped in if necessary, instead of being confined to a wheelchair. After this was done she pressed to have Mrs. L. E. placed in a geri chair instead of a rocker. This change did not satisfy her either. She was further aggravated when Mrs. L. E. failed to express any appreciation for being moved from one chair to another, and left in anger, exasperated by Mrs. L. E.'s lack of response. Running true to form, Mrs. A. C. returned several weeks later and criticized the quality of Mrs. L. E.'s care and contacted the volunteer for help. He had been seeing Mrs. L. E. weekly and met with Mrs. A. C. to talk about her complaints, help her sort out her feelings about Mrs. L. E. and hopefully make the relationship more positive.

Death and Dying

The elderly have a range of perspectives on dying: denying it as a certainty yet living in fear of it; accepting it as God's will and at his discretion; fearing it as a personal annihilation; anticipating it as a release from excruciating pain; and suffering and accepting it as nature completing the life cycle. Frustration, anger, fear and anxiety are likely to be associated with all of these perspectives.

Being with the elderly person, gently extending of yourself to her, is important. This means being available to her if she wants to talk, which she may or may not want to do. Sometimes the dying person is most interested in the physical presence of a trusted, genuinely interested and concerned person. Holding the dying person's hand, stroking her forehead, touching her shoulder may provide meaningful support. A final note, you must appreciate and deal with your own feelings about a dying client and her death. Doing so will make you more helpful to her. Grief and getting over the death of a client may take time, and should be anticipated.

Example: Mrs. S.

Mrs. S. was a victim of progressive cancer, who was moved from her apartment to a nursing home, to a hospital, and back to the nursing home. The last move was made with the recognition that her end was near.

As the volunteer entered the unit, a nursing assistant told him that Mrs. S. was dying. He entered her room, where she was lying on her side, breathing rapidly and perspiring profusely. He greeted her and extended his hand to her, which she slowly grasped. After holding it for several moments, he sat down but continued to hold her hand, and asked, "May I do anything for you?"

She shook her head. However, several minutes later she raised her head and attempted to speak, but could not. She repeated this several times during the hour, but was never able to articulate her interest. After one of these efforts the volunteer stood and stroked her forehead, and then sat back down. She searched his eyes beseechingly, nodded her head, then closed her eyes.

She lay curled up and austere in the meagerly furnished room; her grey hair was combed into smooth order and made even more pronounced by her excessive perspiration. The sheet was folded neatly under her chin and stood in stark contrast to her pain-stricken face.

She went into a coma about an hour later and died shortly thereafter.

In a dream that night the volunteer walked ever so cautiously as he approached a clearing in a dark woods. Its eeriness played upon and enhanced his already-existing fear. As he reached the clearing he saw Mrs. S. lying in her hospital bed, but strangely, it was in a helicopter and it was lifting above its landing pad, which curiously was her room in the nursing home. Though moving upward it was without a pilot. Mrs. S., with her head slightly raised from the pillow, called desperately to be rescued. The volunteer rushed forward but his effort was to no avail as the helicopter had moved aloft, leaving him in a whirling debris of dust, grass and smoke.

Surprisingly, the volunteer was able to hear Mrs. S.'s calling above the roar of the helicopter. Only as the aircraft continued to gain altitude did her cries fade. Soon the helicopter was a small object in the sky and the volunteer left the clearing and walked back through the woods, and as he reached its darkest point, he jerked back with a gasp as a bird darted from a bush, flapping its wings and then flew into the sky.

Process: Patience, Detail, and Giving Things Time

Giving the client the time and opportunity to look back into her life, particularly the detail of significant experiences, requires patience. The person's unique manner of unfolding the pages of her life may be by starts and stops, circumventions, hesitancies, resistances, repetitions, and sometimes suspicions. Information may come directly and with exceptional candor, at least parts of it, or it may come indirectly, covered, and by illusions. Major dramas may be presented once and dealt with in terms of expression and resolution, or they may be presented in part denied, and emerge again at a later time. Such dramas may include the choice of a spouse, death of a parent, relationship to a spouse, courtship of a spouse, an academic experience. Whether dealt with in total or in parts, she will consider various facets of the experience and perhaps attempt to connect it to previous and subsequent events and finally to incorporate it all into her overall life experience.

Your approach and technique guide the elderly person's delving into her present and past, help her consider the events clearly and piece them together, and gain a better understanding of her life. As has been indicated, the delving is dynamic rather than orderly. Though overly systematic in terms of how work typically proceeds with the elderly, a brief outline follows.

1. **Making Contact.** It may seem obvious, yet making meaningful contact with the elderly person is basic and foremost, and it may not be easy. Meaningful contact implies mental and emotional connecting with her, not just a cheery greeting and light chitchat. The client must feel you are present for her best behalf, and you must know she feels this. An extended handshake at the beginning and the end of the visit, being patient and taking time during the visit, should communicate empathy, friendship, support, affirmation and fairness. Clear, which often includes slow, explanation of the interview procedures must be stated and include sufficient opportunity for the elderly person to ask questions and discuss her concerns.

2. **Encouraging Expression and Listening.** After making contact with the elderly person, your tasks are as follows: encourage the client to express herself as openly as she can; listen carefully, patiently, and with an ear for the relevance of what she says, and does not say. A bit of teaching about the procedures for the visits should be done; queries must be answered; information should be sought; reassurance must be offered; and above all, you must care and listen. Kindness, affirmation and trust should be apparent.

3. **Reviewing, Clarifying, Focusing.** These tasks may be viewed as a part of listening, but also as distinct tasks by themselves. They ask the client to review, particularly to reconsider, an experience or several experiences for their clarity, significance and relationships, and in the process give the client insight into her situation. Feelings that are part and parcel of the elderly person's recollections should always be brought into play, but very carefully because of their probable volatility.

4. **Deciding the What, How and When of Responding.** These tasks run throughout all of the visiting because you are always deciding "What is going on?" "What does this, that or the other

thing really mean?" "How are things progressing?" "How can I help the process?" "What is the client's condition?" Inquiries, simply stated, to the client on these matters may keep you informed, at least modestly, and in turn you should tell the client how you understand what she has been telling you.

Telling the client how you understand her may include reflecting back to her a different interpretation of events than she may be aware of, or even may have denied. The "What" of your response is typically grounded in what the elderly person has said, and perhaps in part on what she has consistently skipped over. At any rate, she must be given the opportunity to respond, to clarify, accept or reject whatever is under consideration. There are variations on the "How," but given the sensitivity of the client, gentleness and questions rather than confrontation are in order. Further, a sense of humor, an easy manner combined with genuineness will help communicating with the client and in handling the "How" of the matter. The "When" to intervene is a highly subjective matter. Generally, you must take your time, appreciating the client's psychology—how she is feeling, what she is dealing with in considering the various aspects of her life. Her readiness to accept anything from you, especially anything foreign to her view of things, is key. This suggests you cannot be quick to offer opinions or make suggestions, not until she has told her full story, has reflected on it and considered it herself. Even then you must go slowly in offering any special meaning to her thoughts.

5. **Returning to Encourage Expression and Listening**. The client will usually respond to your questions, suggestions, and an occasional reformulation of her views, if appropriately said and timed. Your response then becomes the new focus as she re-engages and you encourage, listen, review, clarify, focus and employ related techniques, not only to stimulate and deal with new substance but also to be alert to previously left but unresolved matters.

6. **Summarization and Termination**. This item has already been discussed earlier in the text. However, an additional consideration pertains to you. It is the necessity for you to examine how you feel about the termination—for example,

might you feel frustrated, sad, relieved, or ambivalent. And you must consider whether any of these possibilities was stimulated by some change in the elderly person's circumstance, such as moving, dying, or having received maximum benefit from the association. Your self-examination is not only important for the immediate circumstance, but also for your future work.

V
Coping With Stress

Even though working with the elderly, becoming involved in their lives offers many satisfactions, it can be taxing and generate stress. Here are several points to manage the stress.

- Recognize that visiting with elderly persons, becoming acquainted with their problems, and helping them struggle with them is likely to produce stress and some personal discomfort. This goes with the work as much as the satisfactions and joys. Do not deny it. Think about it. Choose how to deal with it.
- How to recognize the presence of stress:
  • Excessive worry about the clients
  • Chronic tiredness
  • Tendency to forget appointments with clients
  • Muscle tension
  • Unexplained anxiety or anxiety specifically about calling on the clients
  • Nervousness, sleeplessness
  • General body complaints
- How to handle the stress:
  • Assuming the presence of stress yet a lack of clarity about its origins, you might consider the various facets of your personal affairs in addition to your work with the elderly. Consider family matters, relationships to friends, and so on. Try to be open and non-defensive.
  • Share your thoughts and feelings with others. Talk with your supervisor at the agency, if you are related to one. Also, talk with a family member, or friend, give yourself a chance to regroup and to continue working, perhaps in a different manner.

- Respect personal limits. If you do not, you may become so distraught you cannot be the kind of helper that you want to be.
- Learn to express anxiety, depressed feelings and other upset feelings. They are a part of life, though usually denied or otherwise covered up.
- Choose a "safety-valve" activity—swimming, walking, singing, working—to discharge tension and reset feelings.
- Try not to get down. Remain in charge of yourself and your life. Take an active approach to improve your mood. Enlarge your activities.
- Discover new creative outlets, such as hobbies, skills or interests.
- Remember that along with expressing your various feelings, it is okay to cry. Crying is a very human expression, especially to relieve sadness.
- Stay in touch with friends; involve yourself.
- If you have not already done so, work on developing a sense of humor and realism. Try to laugh at yourself, if such is warranted. Try to be realistic in your expectations and your evaluation of your work.
- Appreciate what you can change and what you cannot.
- Take satisfaction from your contribution.
- Appreciate and value yourself.

VI
Report Writing

Report writing fulfills, at least in part, the task of monitoring the condition and care of the aged person, and conveys your observations and work to the supervisor of the case, for example, a social worker or a guardian. It must be thorough and clear and must cover the client's condition and the quality of the facility's service.

On the Client:

A number of areas must be covered on the client.

1. *Mobility.* Can she walk, unassisted by another person or some physical device, and if she can, how far can she walk? The latter point must consider her strength or frailty. She may be limited to a wheel or geri chair, or perhaps confined to bed or a sofa.
2. *Vigor.* How much energy, strength and vigor does she have? If not at all vigorous, then in what degree of weakness and feebleness is she?
3. *Personal Appearance.* Does she stand erectly? Are her eyes bright? Is her complexion even and fresh looking? Is she clean, neat, and appropriately dressed and groomed? Are her fingernails trimmed and clean? Does she smell okay? Does she show any signs of neglect or abuse, or complain of such?
4. *Mood.* Is she happy and satisfied? Is she even tempered and matter-of-fact? Does she tend to be flat, uninspired and on the down side? Might she be sad, despondent, deeply depressed? Is she anxious and fearful? Is she impulsive and hysterical? Are there any marked swings in her mood, from one extreme to another? How does she feel—generally, okay, that is quite well, quite satisfied, happy, at ease; or at loose ends, bored, distressed, or perhaps in pain?

5. *Thinking.* Is it clear, logical and rational? Is any confusion present? Is there any loss of memory functioning—short term, long term, both? Is she able to converse meaningfully? Does she have any peculiar ideas? Is she suspicious?

What is the content or substance of her conversation? If it consists of reminiscences of her earlier life, about what time period does she speak and what is her specific area of interest? What emotions did she attach to the topics of her conversation? Are there any relationships between recollections of earlier experiences and current circumstances?

6. *Relationships.* Does she relate to others openly, candidly, spontaneously? Or is she reluctant, resistive, perhaps hostile? Is she typically trusting or to the contrary? Is she able to relate to others? Or does she tend to be a loner? Is she easily angered at the slightest provocation?

7. *Health.* In addition to your making observations about her appearance and asking her about how she feels, what does the charge nurse say about her condition? What do the medical records show?

On the Facility:

You also must report the quality of care offered by the facility. The following topics should be considered.

1. *Interpersonal Relations.* Do the staff relate to the client in a patient, encouraging, caring way? Or in some other manner: Curt? Incidental? Casual?

2. *Program.* Does the facility's program offer the client medical and nursing care, arts and crafts, physical therapy, a beauty shop, discussion groups, social work counseling, speech therapy, etc.?

Example of Report Writing: Mrs. V. H.

The volunteer found Mrs. V. H. reclining in her geri chair when he arrived. She was clean, neatly dressed and groomed. Her fingernails were trimmed and clean. Her complexion, though pale, was not different than on previous weeks.

Her mood was even and generally positive. However, it changed as she contemplated her major concern: despair over physical disabilities resulting from a stroke.

Her bodily movements were severely limited because of the stroke, which had paralyzed her right side and confined her to a geri chair.

She had attended bingo the previous week and happily reported that she won one card. This was the second week she had elected this activity. She continued to read her weekly home town paper and *The Washington Post*. She did not pursue any other reading (e.g., magazines or books) beyond that, though she had been encouraged to do it.

Her thinking was clear and generally rational. The paranoid ideas which had been expressed the previous week of others plotting to steal her personal belongings and keep her from participating in the home's activities were not mentioned. Instead, she wondered why she could not walk. She said, "When I came here about a year ago, I could walk. And now I can't." Though she also said, "I have one side of me that works, my left side, my left arm and leg work, but not my right ones," she did not relate that to her stroke, nor was she immediately aware that she had had one.

The volunteer attempted to have her infer a stroke from her symptoms. Rather than saying, "You had a stroke and these are some of the after-effects," an explanation she very likely would have rejected, he ventured, "How do you understand it?"

She responded with, "I just don't know, and I've been thinking about it."

"And what have your thoughts been?"

She shook her head.

"And what have you concluded?"

She did not carry it further. "I've just been thinking."

"Mull it over and share what you think about it. It probably was something that happened to you. Something in the past."

Mrs. V. H. nodded her head but did not say anything further.

The volunteer continued, "You see others here in the same condition."

Mrs. V. H. nodded.

"And what might have happened to them?"

Mrs. V. H. shook her head, suggesting she did not want to pursue it further.

"Okay, think it over, and let's pick it up when you're ready."

She continued to be withdrawn and did not relate to the other patients.

Neither the charge nurse nor the medical record reported any changes in her condition.

The place was clean and the staff was friendly, and after spending about forty-five minutes in the home, the volunteer left.

VII
Ethics and the Volunteer

General Considerations

Working with the elderly obviously involves ethical matters—morals, duties, rules of conduct. Generally, these connect to philosophic ideas. Two philosophical ideas will be considered.

Strawson[1] suggests there are "ideal pictures of life" that must be considered in thinking about human relations. These pictures urge persons to love and serve one another; to strive for personal honor and high mindedness; to be humble; and to work cooperatively for the welfare of all.

Continuing with philosophical ideas, Hart's[2] "truisms" are very different. They consider the world as it is, not how it might be. His truisms hold that humans are vulnerable. They are subject to being hurt, even while having defenses against such. Further, humans are only approximate in equality, limited in their altruism and are somewhere being noble and mean—all of which require institutions of protection.

The application of these ideas to volunteerism is that codes must indicate what should be (the ideal), being mindful of what is (the real); all in the realm of techniques of practice and quality of service.

Specific Considerations

Though an ethical code for volunteers is necessary, it may seem lacking in logic to consider such. You give time, skill and patience out of the "goodness" of your heart. Why speak to you about ethical issues? Further, it could be said that you come to "do" good, not to talk about it. Why raise matters of principle with you? You want to "get on" with your work. Why

---

[1] Strawson, P. F. *Freedom and Resentment*. London: Methuen, 1974.

[2] Hart, H. *Concept of Law*. Clarendon, NJ: Clarendon, 1961.

hold you up to consider academic items? The agencies that engage you may think the same way.

However, ethics for volunteers is warranted to help you appreciate the scope and complexity of your job and to note that good intentions are not enough. Basically, you are asked to reflect on yourself, that is, be introspective, and in some instances be self-critical. In addition, you must prepare yourself to work with the elderly and remain a "student" of your work. Lastly, you must respect the dignity and worth of elderly persons as part of humanitarianism and democratic ideals.

Ethical guidelines for volunteers involve their supervisors as well. However, that is not treated here. A preliminary code for volunteers includes:

1. Assume only those tasks for which you have competence.
2. Seek continuing education to enhance your competence.
3. Determine the kind and amount of supervision and technical consultation you require.
4. Sketch the goals and procedures of your work with clients and do so at the outset. Include input from your supervisor, and review them with your clients periodically and modify if indicated.
5. Do not discriminate because of race, color, religion, age, sex and natural ancestry.
6. Do not gratify your needs at the expense of the client.
7. Be aware of and support the client's network of friends and relatives.
8. Be cognizant and help the client deal with various aspects of her life— physical, mental, social, economic, and spiritual—within your realm of competence.
9. Protect the privacy of the client and use responsibly the information that is gained from the client and others associated with her.
10. Work in the best interest and welfare of the client.
11. Advise the client about the boundaries of your relationship—off hours and emergency availability, vacation coverage, conditions of continuation and termination.
12. Appreciate the competence and obligations of the care personnel and institution caring for the client.[3]

---

[3] For a thorough review of philosophical ideas as they pertain to ethics, see: Rosenbaum, M. (ed.). *Ethics and Values in Psychotherapy: A Guidebook.* New York: The Free Press, 1982.

Appendix A

Resources

Organizations concerned with the elderly typically offer information, technical assistance, consultation, and publications on activities and programs. Also, they hold conventions, meetings, conduct training and concern themselves with policy and legislative matters.

Specifically for Volunteers

American Society of Directors of
    Volunteer Services
American Hospital Association
One N. Franklin
Chicago, IL 60606
(312) 422-3939

Association For Volunteer
    Administration
P.O. Box 4584
Boulder, CO 80306
(303) 541-0238

National Assembly of Voluntary
    Health and Social Welfare
    Organizations
1319 F St. NW, Ste. 601
Washington, DC 20004
(202) 347-2080

Points of Light Foundation
1737 H St. NW
Washington, DC 20006
(202) 223-9186

Retired and Senior Volunteer Program
1201 New York Ave. NW
Washington, DC 20525
(202) 606-5000

International Voluntary Service
Rte. 2 Box 506
Crozet, VA 22932
(804) 823-1826

National Self-Help Clearinghouse
25 W. 43rd St., Room 620
New York, NY 10036-7406
(212) 354-8525

Senior Companion Program
2900 Newton St. NE
Washington, DC 20018
(202) 529-8701

Volunteers In Service To America
1100 Vermont Ave. NW, Ste. 8100
Washington, DC 20525
(202) 606-4845

General Resources

Aging in America
1500 Pelham Pkwy. S.
Bronx, NY 10461
(718) 824-4004

American Association of Homes and
Services For the Aging
901 E St. NW, Ste. 500
Washington, DC 20004-2037
(202) 783-2242

American Association of Retired
Persons (AARP)
601 E St. NW
Washington, DC 20049
(202) 434-2277

American Society On Aging
833 Market St., Ste. 511
San Francisco, CA 94103-1824
(415) 974-9600

Association of Brethren Care Givers
1451 Dundee Ave.
Elgin, IL 60120
(847) 742-5100

Black, Indian, Hispanic, and Asian
Women In Action
122 W. Franklin Ave., Ste. 306
Minneapolis, MN 55404
(612) 870-1193

Catholic Charities USA
1731 King St., Ste. 200
Alexandria, VA 22314
(703) 549-1390

Children of Aging Parents
1609 Woodbourne Rd.
Levittown, PA 19057-1511
(215) 945-6900

Ebenezer Society
2722 Park Ave. S.
Minneapolis, MN 55407
(612) 879-1400

Episcopal Society for Ministry on
Aging
323 Wyndotte St.
Bethlehem, PA 18015
(610) 868-5400

Grandparents Anonymous
1924 Beverly
Sylvan Lake, MI 48320
(810) 682-8384

Grandparents Raising Grandchildren
P.O. Box 104
Colleyville, TX 76034
(817) 577-0435

Grandparents Rights Organization
104 W. Long Lake Rd. #250
Bloomfield Hills, MI 48301
(810) 646-7191

Gray Panthers
P.O. Box 21477
Washington, DC 20009-9477
(202) 466-3132

Hispanic American Geriatrics Society
1 Cutts Rd.
Durham, NH 03824-3102
(603) 868-5757

National Association For Home Care
519 C Street NW
Stanton, Park, Washington, DC 20002
(202) 547-7424

National Association For Lesbian and
   Gay Gerontology
1853 Market St.
San Francisco, CA 94103
(415) 626-7000

National Association For Senior Living
   Industries
184 Duke of Gloucester St.
Annapolis, MD 21401-2523
(410) 263-0991

National Association of Area Agencies
   On Aging
1112 16th St. NW, Ste. 100
Washington, DC 20036
(202) 296-8130

National Association of Nutrition and
   Aging Services Programs
2675 44th St. SW, Ste. 305
Grand Rapids, MI 49509
(616) 531-9909

National Association of State Units On
   Aging
1225 Eye St. NW, Ste. 725
Washington, DC 20005
(202) 898-2578

National Caucus And Center on the
   Black Aged
1424 K St. NW
Washington, DC 20005
(202) 637-8400

National Center On Rural Aging
409 3rd St. SW, Ste. 200
Washington, DC 20024
(202) 479-6683

National Citizens' Coalition For
   Nursing Home Reform
1224 M St. NW, Ste. 301
Washington, DC 20005-5183
(202) 393-2018

National Council of Jewish Women
53 W. 23rd St.
New York, NY 10010
(212) 645-4048

National Council of Negro Women
1667 K St. NW, Ste. 700
Washington, DC 20006
(202) 659-0006

National Council of Senior Citizens
1331 F St. NW
Washington, DC 20004-1171
(202) 347-8800

National Council On The Aging
409 Third St. SW, Ste. 200
Washington, DC 20024
(202) 479-1200

National Hispanic Council On Aging
2713 Ontario Rd. NW
Washington, DC 20009
(202) 265-1288

National Hospice Organization
1901 N. Moore St., Ste. 901
Arlington, VA 22209
(703) 243-5900

National Indian Council On Aging
City Centre, Ste. 510-W
6400 Uptown Blvd. NW
Albuquerque, NM 87110
(505) 883-3302

National Institute on Aging
Information Office
9000 Rockville Pike
Bethesda, MD 20205
(301) 496-1752

National Senior Citizens Law Center
777 S. Figueroa, Ste. 4320
Los Angeles, CA 90017
(213) 236-3890

North American Association of Jewish
Homes and Housing for the Aging
10830 N. Central Expwy., Ste. 150
Dallas, TX 75231-1022
(214) 696-9838

Theos Foundation
322 Blvd. of the Allies, Ste. 105
Pittsburgh, PA 15222-1919
(412) 471-7779

Sources for Particular Concerns

Alcoholics Anonymous
General Service Office of AA
Box 459, Grand Central Station
New York, NY 10163
(212) 870-3400

Alzheimer's Disease and Related
Disorders Association
919 North Michigan Ave., Ste. 1000
Chicago, IL 60611
(800) 272-3900

Narcotics Anonymous
World Service Office
16155 Wyndotte St.
Van Nuys, CA 91406
(818) 780-3951

National Council on Alcoholism
12 W. 21st St.
New York, NY 10010
(212) 206-6770

Older Women's League
666 11th St. NW, Ste. 700
Washington, DC 20001
(202) 783-6686

Sex Information and Education Council
Of United States
130 W. 42nd St., Ste. 350
New York, NY 10036-7901
(212) 819-9770

Widowed Persons
601 E. St. NW
Washington, DC 20049
(202) 434-2260

Appendix B

MEDICATIONS FOR MENTAL HEALTH
A GUIDE FOR CONSUMERS, FAMILIES, FRIENDS. BOARD AND CARE HOMES, & CAREGIVERS

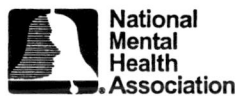

National
Mental
Health
Association

1021 Prince Street, Alexandria, VA 22314-2971 • Phone (703) 684-7722 • Fax (703) 684-5968 • TTY (800) 433-5959 • www.nmha.org
Monty Moeller, Chair of the Board • Michael M. Faenza, President and CEO

Prescription medications are helpful in reducing symptoms in people suffering with a mental illness. As with any medication, there are precautions to be taken, and careful monitoring is needed to reduce any risk and maximize the benefits of medications. It is important for you and others to be familiar with how these medications are used.

HOW DO MEDICATIONS FOR MENTAL HEALTH WORK?
Some mental illnesses are due to chemical imbalances in the brain. These chemicals are neurotransmitters. They are the messengers within the brain which enable communication between different areas of the brain and the body. When there are disturbances in the functioning of these neurotransmitters, the communication system in the brain can be disrupted. Medications can correct the imbalance of these chemicals in the brain and restore healthy neurotransmitter communication. Medications can reduce the symptoms of an acute attack and prevent recurring illness.

TELL YOUR DOCTOR IF YOU:
* Have had allergic reactions to drugs or food
* Are taking any other medications
* Are pregnant or breast-feeding
* Have diabetes, kidney, liver or heart disease
* Are on a special diet or taking any supplements
* Smoke or drink alcohol
* Stop taking the prescribed medications
* Feel side effects

83

There are 5 major categories of mental health medications: Lithium, anti-anxiety, anti-psychotic, anti-depressant, and stimulant medications. Ask your doctor what category of medications you are taking.

Remember:
- Take all medications only as prescribed by your doctor.
- Check your prescription with your pharmacist.
- Know your medication.
- Follow directions and read the label carefully.
- Store medications properly.
- Never stop medications on your own.
- Ask about special precautions.
- Find out about possible side effects.
- Keep your doctor informed about any side effects you may have.

If you have any questions or problems call your doctor, therapist and/or pharmacist.

PLEASE NOTE: **These medications should only be prescribed by your doctor.**

ANTI-DEPRESSANTS

Generic Names	Brand Names
Amitriptyline	Elavil, Endep
Amoxapine	Asendin
Desipramine	Norpramin
Doxepine	Sinequan, Adapin
Fluoxetine	Prozac
Imipramine	Tofranil
Maprotiline	Ludiomil
Nortriptyline	Aventyl, Pamelor
Paroxetine	Paxil
Phenylzine sulfate	Nardil
Protriptyline	Vivactil
Sertraline	Zoloft
Trazodone	Desyrel
Buproprion	Wellbutrin

WHAT ARE THEY USED FOR? Anti-depressant medication may be used to treat certain kinds of depression: depressed mood, loss of interest, lack of pleasure, decreased need for sleep and food. These drugs treat depression by supplying some of the missing chemicals that make you feel well and happy. Anti-depressants can help you come out of the depression and help prevent its recurrence.

SIDE EFFECTS FOR TRICYCLICS: Dizziness, sleepiness, dry mouth, low blood pressure, blurred vision and constipation may occur. These effects often decrease in 1 to 2 weeks.

PRECAUTIONS:
- Anti-depressants may take 2 weeks or more to take effect.
- Avoid barbiturates and alcohol.
- Do not operate a car or machinery if feeling sleepy.
- If you are pregnant or breast feeding, consult your doctor about the risks of using anti-depressants.
- Stopping these medications may result in relapse.
- There may be dietary precautions while taking MAO inhibitors.

ANTI-PSYCHOTICS

Generic Names	Brand Names
Chlorpromazine	Thorazine
Fluphenazine	Prolixin
Haloperidol	Haldol
Loxapine	Loxitane
Mesoridazine	Serejail
Molindone	Moban
Perphenazine	Trilafon
Thioridazine	Mellaril
Thiothixene	Navane
Trifluoperazine	Stelazine
Clozapine	Clozaril*
Risperidone	Risperdal*

*Atypical anti-psychotic (ask your doctor about side effects)

WHAT ARE THEY USED FOR? Anti-psychotic medications are used to treat schizophrenia. This disease
causes distorted thinking, confusion of reality and fantasy, and hallucinations. Anti-psychotics can reduce or stop these experiences.

WHAT DO THEY DO? Anti-psychotics treat schizophrenia by supplying some of the chemicals that make you feel organized and concentrated. Anti-psychotic meds help reduce excitability, confusion, and withdrawal. They improve your ability to communicate, to separate reality from fantasy and control hallucinations.

SIDE EFFECTS: Sleepiness, dry mouth, dizziness, blurred vision, rapid heart beat, stuffy nose and constipation may occur. Also, muscle spasms, restlessness, muscle stiffness, trembling, and shaking hands may occur. These effects often disappear in 1 to 2 weeks. Tardive dyskinesia, which is an involuntary movement of the face or mouth, may occur while taking anti-psychotics. It is sometimes irreversible.

PRECAUTIONS: The same precautions apply as with anti-anxiety medications; however, anti-psychotics are not addictive.

ANTI-ANXIETY
Benzodiazepines

Alprazolam	Xanax
Clonazepam	Klonopin
Chlorazapate	Tranxene
Chlordiazepoxide	Librium
Diazepam	Valium
Flurazepam	Dalmane
Lorazepam	Ativan
Oxazepam	Serax
Temazepam	Restoril

Non-Benzodiazepines

Buspirone HCI*	Buspar
Zolpidem	Ambien

*Buspirone lacks sedative and muscle relaxant effects.

WHAT ARE THEY USED FOR? These medications may be used to treat anxiety (an unreasonable state of tension and uneasiness, not ordinary tension), insomnia (difficulty sleeping), tension, and sometimes muscle spasms.

WHAT DO THEY DO? Anti-anxiety medications treat anxiety by supplying some of the missing chemicals that make you feel relaxed and calm. They can provide mild sedation and relief from tension and anxiety.

SIDE EFFECTS: Sleepiness, slurred speech, confusion, headaches, nausea, breathing difficulties (rarely), nervousness, or excitement may occur.

PRECAUTIONS:
- Avoid barbiturates and alcohol if taking these meds. The combination can be **DEADLY.**
- Do not operate a car or machinery until you are sure that the medication does not adversely affect you.
- If you are pregnant or breast feeding consult your doctor about possible risks.
- If taken for a long period of time, these medications can be addictive.

LITHIUM - Generic name - Lithium carbonate/Brand name - Eskalith, Lithane.

WHAT IS IT USED FOR? Lithium may be used to treat mania (overly self-confident, reckless, uncontrollable, sleepless, and excited), or manic depression (alternating between mania and depression).

WHAT DOES IT DO? Lithium adjusts some of the chemicals that make you feel happy and confident, stabilizes your mood, and controls highs and lows. It helps prevent mania and manic-depression from recurring. Lithium may take 4-14 days to take effect.

SIDE EFFECTS: During the first 5 days of treatment it may cause nausea, cramps, thirst, and muscle weakness. 5 to 6 weeks after treatment has begun muscle weakness, fatigue, weight gain and slightly impaired memory may occur. Other more serious effects include diarrhea, vomiting, severe shakiness, and lack of coordination.

PRECAUTIONS:
- Be aware of your salt intake. A low salt concentration in your body can cause fatigue, slurred speech and trembling. In severe cases, coma or death may result.
- Blood tests are necessary to make sure Lithium levels are safe and effective.
- If you are pregnant or breast feeding, consult your doctor about possible risks.
- Stopping this medication may result in relapse.

Note: Medication for children was striken from this technical memorandum because of its irrelevance to the elderly.

General References

AARP (1994). *A Reminiscence Training Kit.* Washington, D.C.: AARP.

American Medical Association (1992). *Diagnostic and Treatment Guidelines on Elder Abuse and Neglect.* Chicago: The Association.

Atchley, R. C. (1988). *Social Forces and Aging.* Belmont, CA: Wadesworth Publishing Co.

Benjamin, A. (1981). *The Helping Interview.* Boston: Houghton Mifflin Co.

Berghorn, F. J., and Schafer, D. E. (1987). "Reminiscence Intervention in Nursing Homes: What and Who Changes?" *International Journal of Aging and Human Development,* 24(2), 113-127.

Butler, R. N. (1975). *Why Survive? Being Old in America.* New York: Harper and Row, Publishers,

Butler, R. N. and Lewis, M. I. (1982). *Aging and Mental Health.* St. Louis: C.V. Mosby Co.

Curran, J. J. (1990). *Nursing Homes: What You Need to Know.* Baltimore: Attorney General Office, Consumer Protection Division.

Erickson, E. H., Erickson, J. M., and Kivnick, H. Q. (1986). *Vital Involvement in Old Age.* New York: Norton.

Esser, A. H., and S. D. Liacey (1989). *Mental Illness: A Homecare Guide.* New York: John Wiley.

Fitzgerald, H. (1994). *The Mourning Handbook*. New York: Simon and Schuster.

Hollis, F. and Woods, M.E. (1981). *Casework: A Psychosocial Therapy*. New York: Random House.

Horne, J. (1985). *Caregiving: Helping an Aging Loved One*. Greenview, IL: Scott, Foresman.

Kastenbaum, R. and Aisenberg, R. (1976). *The Psychology of Death*. New York: Springer Publishing Co.

Klein, D. and P. Wender (1993). *Understanding Depression: A Complete Guide to Its Diagnosis, Course, and Treatment*. New York: Oxford University Press.

Perlman, M. K. (1979). *Relationship: The Heart of Helping People*. Chicago: University of Chicago Press.

Rosenblatt, P. C., Walsh, R. P. and Jackson, D. A. (1976). *Grief and Mourning in Cross-Cultural Perspective*. New Haven, CN: HRAF Press.

Ross, J. (1994). *Triumph over Fear: A Book of Help and Hope for People with Anxiety, Panic Attacks, and Phobias*. New York: Bantam.

Weber, G. H. (1990). *Geriatric Nursing Assistants*. Westport, Connecticut: Greenwood Press.

Webster, J. D., and Yong, R. A. (1988). "Process Variables of the Life Review: Counseling Implications." *The International Journal of Aging and Human Development*, 26(4), 315-323.

Yudofsky, S.C. et al. (1992). *What You Need to Know about Psychiatric Drugs*. New York: Ballantine.

Zeithin, S. J., Katkin, A. J., Baker, H. C. (1982). *A Celebration of American Family Folklife*. New York: Pantheon.

Index